2nd Edition

Laboratory Manual for Clinical Kinesiology & Anatomy

Lynn S. Lippert, MS, PT
Mt. Hood Community College (Retired)
Gresham, Oregon

Mary Alice Duesterhaus Minor, MS, PT
Clinical Assistant Professor
Clarkson University
Potsdam, New York

F. A. DAVIS COMPANY • Philadelphia

F. A. Davis Company
1915 Arch Street
Philadelphia, PA 19103
www.fadavis.com

Printed in the United States of America

Last digit indicates print number: 10 9 8 7 6 5 4

Acquisitions Editor: Margaret M. Biblis
Manager of Content Development: Deborah J. Thorp
Developmental Editor: Peg Waltner
Art and Design Manager: Carolyn O'Brien
ISBN 10: 0-8036-1375-X
ISBN 13: 978-0-8036-1375-1

Laboratory Manual for Clinical Kinesiology & Anatomy

2nd Edition

To students who desire to understand so as to help others.

MADM

To Kate and Kellen, who succeeded in keeping their promise to remain recognizable members of the human race during their teen years, I wish them success as they find their place in life.

LSL

Preface to Second Edition

This edition of the *Laboratory Manual for Clinical Kinesiology and Anatomy* has several major changes. The addition of several new chapters makes for a closer correlation to *Clinical Kinesiology and Anatomy* 4th ed. by Lynn S. Lippert. Photographs showing hand placement for many palpations are another major change. Each chapter still has three parts, Worksheets to be completed prior to class, Lab Activities to be completed in class, and Post-Lab Questions to be completed after class. We believe that students who complete the Worksheets prior to class will be familiar with the content and prepared to participate during class. The Post-Lab questions provide the student with the opportunity to review the material after class. Although each chapter directs student learning, each chapter is designed to promote active learning. We believe, students actively engaged in their learning are more likely to gain understand and retain what they have learned.

The first seven chapters are devoted to basic information that is then applied in the next 12 chapters dedicated to specific body segments. The final two chapters are devoted to posture and gait. Examining posture provides students with the opportunity to consider the interrelationships of the various body segments. Walking is our preferred method of mobility when performing our activities of daily living. Having an appreciation for the complexity of walking is necessary to be able to examine someone's gait for effectiveness and efficiency.

A note about the photographs is in order. We attempted to show hand placement, bony landmarks, and muscles in the photographs. To do this, the position of the subject and person performing the palpations may have been altered from the desired position to obtain an unobstructed view. Muscles are not always obvious. We chose subjects who represent average individuals and not body builders to more closely resemble what students are likely to find when observing their partners.

Preface to the First Edition

This laboratory manual is designed to complement Lippert's *Clinical Kinesiology for Physical Therapist Assistants,* but it can be used with other textbooks as well. Each chapter of the manual is divided into three parts: Worksheets, Lab Activities, and Post-Lab Questions.

- The Worksheets are designed to assist the student in preparing for the lab session and should be completed by the student prior to class.
- The Lab Activities are designed to be completed in small groups as part of the lab session. The resources needed for the activities are those readily available and are not costly.
- The Post-Lab Questions are to be completed outside the lab sessions as a review.

We attempted to include the same key concepts in each chapter, as applicable, to allow the students to apply those concepts to a new body region.

The focus of the manual is on understanding normal kinesiology, and thus a selection of normal activities has been presented. We believe that students need to understand normal function before they can appreciate the abnormal. For this reason, the chapters on gait and posture, for example, include a general overview of the normal.

Arthrokinetic concepts involving the convex-concave law are included to provide an introduction to basic joint movements. However, by including this material, we do not mean to imply, suggest, or promote the idea that joint mobilization is an entry-level skill for physical therapist assistants. The concept of open-chain versus closed-chain activities, having gained popularity in the last few years, has also been included.

This manual is the result of many years of teaching kinesiology to PTA, OTA, and PT students. The authors test-piloted this version during development with the classes they were teaching. Student participation in lab sessions improved, feedback was positive, and suggestions were incorporated into the final version. We thank our students for their patience and their helpful suggestions.

MADM

LSL

ACKNOWLEDGMENTS

Again I had the privilege and pleasure to work with Lynn Lippert. Her insight and organization kept the project moving forward. In addition to working with Lynn, I worked with my favorite photographer, my daughter Sarah Minor. She had great patience with our requests for another view. I also thank my husband, Scott Minor, for his support during the development of this edition.

MADM

Computer technology has advanced since the creation of the first edition. The computer's ability to crash at inopportune moments makes me extremely grateful to Jon Bridenbaugh for his computer fixing skills. It has been a pleasure to work again with Mary Alice Minor. Her eagle eye saw things I had missed and her ability to find time in a very busy schedule allowed us to complete the project on time. Sal Jepson can never be thanked enough for her wisdom, input, and support. Her original illustrations remain the backbone of this lab manual.

LSL

We thank the people at F. A. Davis for their continued support of this manual. We particularly thank those who worked so diligently with us: Margaret Biblis, Publisher; Deborah J. Thorp, Content Development Manager; and the rest of the production team. We especially thank Peg Waltner, Developmental Editor, for her tenacity and desire to make sure everything was correct. Debbie Van Dover, MEd, PT, Sandy Molhoek, PTA, and Erin Janssens were invaluable for their participation and assistance during the photo shoot. Their efforts made the day successful and enjoyable.

REVIEWERS

Denise Abrams, PT
Chairperson/Professor
Physical Therapist Assistant
    Department
Broome Community College
Binghamton, New York

Debra A. Belcher, PT, DPT
Physical Therapy Assistant
    Department
Sinclair Community College
Dayton, Ohio

Ruth Eccles, PT, MHS, OCS
Coordinator
Physical Therapy Assistant Program
Morton Community College
Cicero, Illinois

Brenda W. Henoch, MPT
Instructor
Physical Therapy Assistant Program
Whatcom Community College
Bellingham, Washington

Amy Murphy, BS
Instructor Specialist
Physical Therapy Assistant Program
Anne Arundel Community College
Arnold, Maryland

Christopher W. O'Brien, MS, ATC
Program Director of Athletic Training
    Education
Health and Physical Education
    Department
Marywood University
Scranton, Pennsylvania

Priscilla Ann Tucker, PT, MA
Program Director
Physical Therapist Assistant Program
Wallace Community College
Dothan, Alabama

CONTENTS

Basic Clinical Kinesiology
and Anatomy

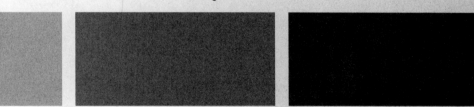

Basic Information

■ ■ ■ Worksheets

Student's Name _____ Date Due _____

Kinesiology is the science that deals with the relationships between anatomical structure and physiological processes that result in human movement. Knowledge of basic kinesiological concepts is fundamental to understanding the stresses placed on joints and joint structures when exercises and functional tasks are performed. Movements of bones affect the motions of joint surfaces in distinct patterns. Interaction between bone movements and the associated joint surface movements can be therapeutic or damaging. Appling fundamental kinesiological concepts correctly is important to achieve desired outcomes.

To examine human movement, several basic definitions used in kinesiology must be understood. These definitions demonstrate the interrelationship between structure and function. Definitions that are necessary for understanding and using the exercises in this laboratory manual are included in Lippert's *Clinical Kinesiology and Anatomy* 4th Edition, Chapter 1. Activities in this chapter will assist in gaining an understanding of these terms and development of other useful skills.

Complete the following questions prior to lab class.

1. Define the following:

   Kinesiology:

   _____

   Biomechanics:

   _____

   Kinetics:

   _____

   Kinematics:

   _____

Observation

Much information about a person is obtained by observation. Methods of observation include the tactile, visual, and auditory senses. The tactile mode of observation is called palpation. Palpation uses the sense of touch to perceive information concerning bony landmarks; crepitus; muscle tone, shape, and size; skin texture and temperature; swelling; tenderness; and pulses. Visual observation uses the sense of sight to perceive information concerning individuals such as how they perform activities of daily living; their gait and movement patterns; and nail, scar, and skin condition. Auditory observation uses the sense of hearing to perceive information such as breath sounds, foot contact during gait, and the sound of a person's voice.

Visual Observations

Practitioners use their eyes to gain information about a person starting at the first meeting. Physical characteristics such as gender, hair and eye color, and height and weight are assessed visually first. Practitioners particularly note how a person moves and the postures assumed. These observations provide a starting point for investigating a person's problems and the developing appropriate interventions.

Auditory Observations

Auditory observations also provide useful information. When a person has an uneven gait pattern, the noise made by the feet contacting the supporting surface can be uneven in volume or rhythm. A person with a respiratory problem often coughs, clears the throat, and may produce sounds such as whizzing. Some sounds, such as lung sounds and blood pressure, require the use of a stethoscope, whereas other sounds are audible without amplification.

Palpation Observations

Usually, fingertips are used when performing palpation. The dorsum of the hand, however, is used to note the temperature of a body area. Knowing how hard to press when performing palpation is important. Too little pressure does not convey enough information from the subject to your fingertips. For example, a bony landmark may not be found because insufficient pressure is used to feel the landmark through the overlying skin and muscle. Too much pressure obliterates the information to be conveyed to your fingertips and can be uncomfortable for the person being palpated. An example of applying too much pressure is when a pulse cannot be felt because excessive pressure occludes the artery. The degree of pressure used during palpation can be learned by guided practice and feedback. Knowing where structures to be palpated are located is an important outcome of studying anatomy and kinesiology.

Estimating Joint Angles

A task often performed during visual observation is estimating the angle of a joint, for example determining the amount of elbow flexion range of motion present. Estimation of joint angle requires having a reference point from which any change or deviation from that point can be determined. The reference point used most often is the anatomical position. Generally joint angles are considered to be zero in the anatomical position. There are a few exceptions such as forearm pronation and supination. A method of learning to estimate joint angle uses the 0°, 45°, 90°, 135°, and 180° positions as reference points. Visualize the face of an analog clock. Visualize the zero position as being when both hands are at the 12 o'clock position, by keeping the hour hand over the 12 and moving the minute hand, various angles can be formed. Placing the minute hand over the 3 forms a 90° angle, over the 6 forms a 180° angle. A point halfway between 12 and 3 forms a 45° angle. A point halfway between 3 and 6 forms a 135° angle.

   Estimating the 0° and 90° positions of a joint is usually easy. Visualize the 0° and 90° positions of the joint being observed. When the actual joint angle is less than 90°, visualize the 45° position, a position halfway between 0° and 90°, and determine if the position being observed is less than, equal to, or greater than 45° and then estimate the angle. When the actual joint angle is greater than 90°, visualize the 135° position, a position halfway between 90° and 180°, and determine if the position being observed is less than, equal to, or greater than 135°, and then estimate the angle.

   Use Figures 1-1A through 1-1E to practice. Figure 1-1A presents a stick figure of an elbow in full extension, meaning the elbow is straight. This position is the 0° angle of elbow flexion

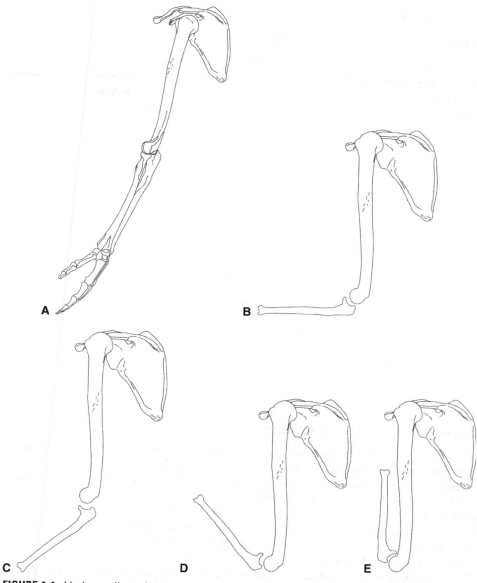

FIGURE 1-1. Various elbow joint positions. *(A)* Full elbow extension, or 0° elbow flexion. *(B)* 90° elbow flexion. *(C)* 45° elbow flexion, the mid-point between 0° and 90° elbow flexion. *(D)* 135° elbow flexion. Calculated by adding an estimated 45° arch (as in C) to the quarter circle that represents 90° (90° + 45° = 135°). *(E)* Hypothetical position of 180° elbow flexion.

or extension. Figure 1-1B represents an elbow in 90° of elbow flexion, such as when a subject has moved from the anatomical position to a position where the palm is parallel to and facing the ceiling. One-quarter of a full circle represents 90°, placing the forearm at a right angle, or perpendicular, to the humerus. When the elbow is halfway between position 0° and 90° of elbow flexion, the elbow joint position is 45°, as in Figure 1-1C. When the elbow is an additional 45° beyond 90° of elbow flexion, the elbow position is 135°, as in Figure 1-1D. Estimate an arc of 45° as in Figure 1-1C, and add it to the quarter-circle position that represents 90° of elbow flexion as in Figure 1-1B (90° + 45° = 135°). For purposes of comparison, 180° of elbow flexion, which should not be possible because of muscle bulk and joint structure, is presented in Figure 1-1E.

2. On the following table:

    A. List some characteristics that can be observed while examining a person.

    B. List which sensory modality is used to perceive the characteristic.

Characteristics	Sense

Joint Movements (Osteokinematics)

In kinesiology, a distinction is made between the movements of bones or limb segments (osteokinematics) and the movements of the joint surfaces at the ends of bones (arthrokinematics). A **limb segment** is considered to be composed of the bones themselves. In the case of elbow flexion, the proximal limb segment would be the humerus and the distal limb segment would be the radius and ulna (forearm). Movement of a limb segment is described by the direction of movement of the bones in space. Naming limb segment movements is standardized by using the **anatomical position** as the starting position. Osteokinematics describes the movements of bones (or limb segments) in space, without regard to the movement of joint surfaces of the bones. For example, in the anatomical position, the forearm limb segment, the radius and ulna, move forward and upward, and the osteokinematics term used to describe this motion is flexion.

3. Examples of osteokinematics include the limb segment movements of flexion and extension (hyperextension), abduction and adduction, and medial and lateral rotation. Review definitions for limb movements given in Lippert's text, *Clinical Kinesiology and Anatomy* 4th Edition, Chapter 1, and then match the following descriptions of motions to the correct term.

    The reference position is the anatomical position unless otherwise indicated. Use each answer only once.

    _____S__ Pulling your scapulae together

    _____E__ Moving your leg toward the midline

    _____L__ Rolling your arm outward

    _____I__ Moving your hand toward the thumb side

    _____J__ Turning your foot inward

    A. Flexion

    B. Extension

    C. Hyperextension

    D. Abduction

    E. Adduction

___O___ Move your arm through a cone-shaped arc

___Q___ Moving your arm across the body at shoulder level

___N___ Moving your hand down the side of your leg

___C___ Shoulder motion during bowling back swing

___G___ Turning your palm posteriorly

___D___ Moving your arm out to the side

___B___ The position of the knee in standing

___F___ The position of the forearm in anatomical position

___A___ Moving the thigh forward and upward

___H___ Synonymous with wrist adduction

___P___ Moving your arm outward from 90° shoulder abduction

___K___ Moving your foot outward

___R___ Moving your scapulae away from the midline

___M___ Turning your arm inward

A. Supination

B. Pronation

C. Ulnar deviation

D. Radial deviation

E. Inversion

F. Eversion

G. Lateral rotation

M. Medial rotation

I. Lateral bending

J. Circumduction

Q. Horizontal abduction

N. Horizontal adduction

O. Protraction

P. Retraction

4. On the drawing, identify linear motion and angular motion.

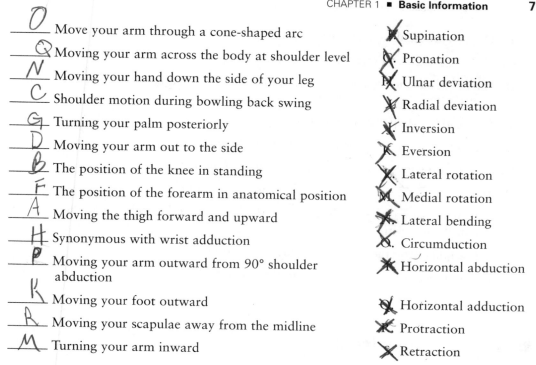

FIGURE 1-2. Bicycle rider.

5. Using the following descriptive terms, fill in the blanks to complete the sentences. Terms may be used more than once.

Medial   Superior   Proximal   Superficial   Anterior
Lateral   Inferior   Distal   Deep   Posterior

A. The tibia is the __Anterior__ bone of the lower leg, and the fibula is the __Posterior__ bone of the lower leg.

B. The ribs are _Inferior_ to the scapula.

C. The _Distal_ end of the humerus is at the elbow joint.

D. The brachialis muscle lies underneath the biceps; therefore, it is _Deep_ to the biceps.

E. The head is _Superior_ to the chest.

F. The _Proximal_ end of the tibia is at the knee joint.

G. The great toe is on the _Medial_ side of the foot.

H. Your eye is _Superior_ and _Lateral_ to your mouth.

I. The radius is on the _Lateral_ side of the forearm, and the ulna is on the _Medial_ side of the forearm.

J. The scapula is on the _posterior_ side of the trunk.

K. The shoulder girdle is _Superior_ to the pelvic girdle.

L. Skin is _Superficial_ to muscle.

■ ■ ■ Lab Activities

Student's Name _____ Date Due _____

1. In a group, students perform the following active motions.

Shoulder:	Flexion	Extension
	Abduction	Adduction
	Horizontal abduction	Horizontal adduction
	Lateral rotation	Medial rotation
Elbow:	Flexion	Extension
Hip:	Flexion	Extension
	Abduction	Adduction
	Lateral rotation	Medial rotation
Knee:	Flexion	Extension

2. Perform the following activities as small groups. Students make note of the speed and distance traveled by each person.

   A. Line students up shoulder to shoulder and instruct them to walk across the room keeping their line straight.

   B. Line students up shoulder to shoulder in the middle of the room and instruct them to walk in a circle with the student on the right end as the pivot or anchor.

   C. Repeat activity B with the student on the left end as the pivot or anchor.

   D. Compare the speed of movement of each student in activities A, B, and C.

   _____

   _____

   E. Compare distance traveled by each student in activities A, B, and C.

   _____

   _____

F. What type of motion is performed in activity A?

_____

G. What type of motion is performed in activities B and C?

_____

3. To practice palpation, use the finger pads of your right index and middle fingers. Place your fingertips lightly on the anterior surface of your left forearm just proximal to the wrist with your left wrist flexed. Extend your left wrist and note the changing sensations in your fingertips as wrist extension causes the tendons of the wrist and finger flexors to become taut. Move your fingertips medially and laterally (side to side) over the wrist and finger flexor tendons making note of the changing sensations as you move over the tendons. Note how lightly you are touching and are able to palpate the changes. Describe what you felt in your right fingers as you palpated.

_____

_____

4. Palpate using your finger pads over the muscles on the lateral aspect of your forearm just distal to the elbow joint. Using light pressure, move your fingers over the area. Describe what you feel. (Hard, soft, firm).

_____

_____

5. With your finger pads over the muscles on the lateral aspect of your forearm just distal to the elbow joint, gradually increase the pressure of your palpation until it becomes slightly uncomfortable. Note how much pressure you are using. Patients, particularly those in pain or with fragile tissues, may not tolerate that amount of pressure. Repeat the muscle palpation using your fingertips. What problem may you encounter palpating with your fingertips?

_____

6. Palpate using your finger pads over the dorsal aspect of the elbow. This is a bony area. Describe what you feel.

_____

_____

7. Compare the pressure used to palpate at the wrist, forearm, and elbow. Compare and contrast the sensations you felt at each area.

_____

_____

_____

8. Repeat the previous palpations on your partner. Did you feel the same characteristics as when you palpated yourself? Were you able to adjust your pressure to a comfortable level for your partner while still being able to make the observations you needed?

_____

_____

9. Place the dorsum (back) of your hand on the anterior surface of your partner's foot. Gradually move your hand proximally to just proximal to the knee joint. Describe the temperature of your partner's lower extremity.

   _____

   _____

10. Practice the following observation and palpation skills on at least two partners.
    A. Palpate the biceps brachii muscle belly and tendons. The biceps brachii is on the anterior surface of the humerus. Palpate the relaxed muscle, and then, while your partner is contracting the muscle.
       1) Describe how you used your hands to palpate (e.g., fingertips, light pressure).

          _____

          _____

       2) Describe the difference you palpated between the muscle relaxed and the muscle contracted. Did what you palpated feel any different when the biceps muscle was contracting?

          _____

          _____

       3) Did contracting the muscle help you to find the tendon?

          _____

          _____

    B. Palpate the medial and lateral epicondyles of the humerus—bony projections on the medial and lateral sides at the elbow.
       1) Describe how you used your hands to palpate.

          _____

          _____

       2) Describe what you felt.

          _____

          _____

    C. Palpate the patellar tendon—first, with the quadriceps muscle relaxed, and then, with your partner contracting the muscle. The patellar tendon is on the anterior of the knee just below the patella (kneecap).
       1) Describe how you used your hands to palpate.

          _____

          _____

       2) Describe what you felt.

          _____

          _____

3) Did the tendon feel any different when the quadriceps muscle was contracting?

_____

_____

4) If you felt a difference in the tendon between the noncontracted state and the contracted state, describe the difference.

_____

_____

5) Did contracting the muscle help you to find the tendon?

_____

_____

D. Palpate your partner's pulse at the radial artery. The radial artery is palpated on the anterior surface of the forearm on the lateral side.

1) Describe how you used your hands to palpate.

_____

_____

2) Describe how the pulse felt—weak, strong, regular, irregular.

_____

_____

E. Palpate the ulnar nerve on the posterior medial aspect of the elbow as the nerve passes just lateral to the medial epicondyle.

1) Describe how you used your hands to palpate the nerve.

_____

_____

2) Describe what you felt.

_____

_____

3) Describe how your partner reacted when you palpated the ulnar nerve with increasing pressure.

_____

_____

F. Posture examination is a visual observation. A person's posture is compared to the normal or ideal posture. Symmetry and deviation from normal posture are noted. Because you have not studied posture yet, compare the second of the following two postures to the first, making note of major changes. Example: In the preferred standing position, your partner shifts a major portion of body weight to the left leg.

1) Observe your partner while he or she is standing erect with weight distributed equally on both feet, which are placed approximately 4 inches apart with the toes pointed forward.

2) Observe your partner standing in his or her preferred standing posture.

3) Describe any major differences between the two postures.

_____

_____

11. You and your partner can practice estimating joint angles. Begin by placing a full circle goniometer in the following positions and observe the angle created. Place the arms of the goniometer so that they are on top of one another. This is the zero or 360° position. Move one arm of the goniometer to the 90° position, to the 45° position, to the 135° position, and to the 180° position.

Starting with your arms in the anatomical position observe what each of the following positions is like.

A. Assume a position of 90° of shoulder flexion.

B. Next extend your shoulder to 45°, a position halfway between the 0° and 90° positions.

C. Next flex your shoulder to 135°, a position halfway between 90° and 180°.

D. Assume a position of 180° of shoulder flexion.

E. Next use another joint, such as the elbow or knee, and assume the same angles of motion observing what each position is like.

Are you able to assume all positions (0°, 45°, 90°, 135°, and 180°) at the elbow and knee joints?

_____

12. To practice visual observation look at your partner.

A. Describe your partner's physical characteristics such as gender, height, and hair and eye color.

_____

_____

B. Make faces to represent different emotional and physical states such as happy, sad, mad, and in pain. Your partner is to guess which state you are displaying.

13. To practice auditory observations, start with your back to your partner so you cannot see what your partner is doing.

A. While your partner is facing away from you, perform some ADLs such as taking off your shoes, removing your shirt, and walking. Ask your partner to describe what they heard and to tell you what activity you performed.

_____

_____

B. If you know how, take your partner's blood pressure paying particular attention to the sounds rather than the pressure reading.

C. Using a stethoscope, listen to your partner's heart and lungs. Describe the sounds you heard.

_____

_____

14. Perform as many of the following motions as possible in the positions of standing, sitting, supine, and side-lying.

Shoulder girdle:	Elevation and depression Upward and downward rotation	Protraction and retraction
Shoulder:	Flexion, extension, and hyperextension Horizontal abduction and adduction Medial and lateral rotation	Abduction and adduction Circumduction
Elbow:	Flexion and extension	
Forearm:	Supination and pronation	
Wrist:	Flexion and extension Circumduction	Radial and ulnar deviation
Finger:	Flexion and extension	Abduction and adduction
Thumb:	Flexion and extension Opposition	Abduction and adduction
Hip:	Flexion, extension, and hyperextension Medial and lateral rotation	Abduction and adduction Circumduction
Knee:	Flexion and extension	
Ankle:	Dorsiflexion and plantar flexion	Inversion and eversion
Toe:	Extension and flexion	

15. Perform the previously listed movements in random order and have your partner name the movement that you are performing.

■ ■ ■ Post-Lab Questions

Student's Name _____ Date Due _____

After you have completed the Worksheets and Lab Activities, answer the following questions without using your book or notes. When finished, check your answers.

1. List the senses used when observing a person.

_____

_____

2. List at least two structures of the body on the:
   A. Anterior surface:

   Eyes, Nose, patella

   B. Lateral surface:

   Finger nails, elbow

   C. Posterior surface:

   Scapula, Calcaneous, Glut Max

3. Define the following terms:
   A. Kinesiology:

   The study of human Movement

   B. Flexion:

   The distal end towards the proximal

   C. Medial rotation:

   Internal Rotation - or Rotation towards the midline

   D. Osteokinematics:

   The movement of joints or bones

4. List at least two structures of the body that are:
   A. Superior to the waist.

   Cervical Spine, Mandible

   B. Lateral to the sternum.

   Clavical, Humerous

   C. Inferior to the waist.

   Femur, Tarsals

   D. Distal to the elbow.

   Carpals, phalanges

Skeletal System

■ ■ ■ Worksheets

Student's Name _____ Date Due _____

Complete the following questions prior to lab class.

1. Complete the following table indicating if the listed body parts are part of the axial or appendicular skeleton.

Body Part	Axial	Appendicular
Arms		
Head		
Vertebrae		
Lower extremity		

2. Match the following descriptions of bone markings with the correct term. Use each term only once.

M Projection above a condyle

F Rounded projection at the end of a joint

E Hole

A Spongelike space filled with air

K Tube-shaped opening

J Rounded projection beyond a narrow neck portion

N Less prominent ridge

I Large, rounded projection

O Flat articular surface

L Very large projection

H Large depression

G Linear depression

D Ridge

B Small, rounded projection

C Sharp projection

A. Sinus

B. Tubercle

C. Crest

D. Spine

E. Foramen

F. Condyle

G. Groove

H. Fossa

I. Tuberosity

J. Head

K. Meatus

L. Trochanter

M. Epicondyle

N. Line

O. Facet

3. On the drawing (Fig. 2-1), label the parts of a long bone using the terms listed:

Epiphysis   Epiphyseal plate   Diaphysis   Medullary canal
Endosteum   Metaphysis   Periosteum

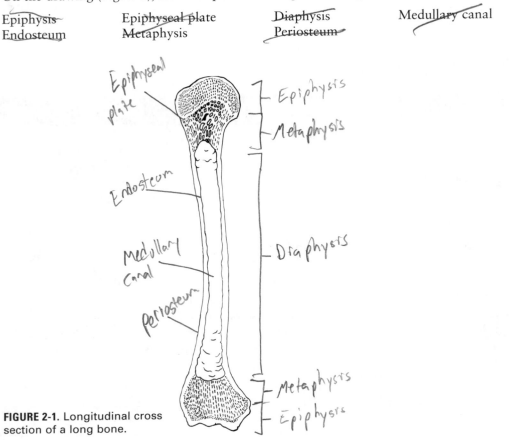

FIGURE 2-1. Longitudinal cross section of a long bone.

4. Complete the following table indicating if the terms are related to compact or cancellous bone.

Characteristic	Compact Bone	Cancellous Bone
Porous and spongy		
Hard and dense		
Covers outside of bone		
Inside portion of bone		

5. Where does longitudinal bone growth occur?

_____

6. What covers most of a bone's surface and what is its purpose?

_____

_____

7. Label the bones in Figure 2-2 using the terms listed below.

Irregular bone   Long bone   Flat bone   Short bone

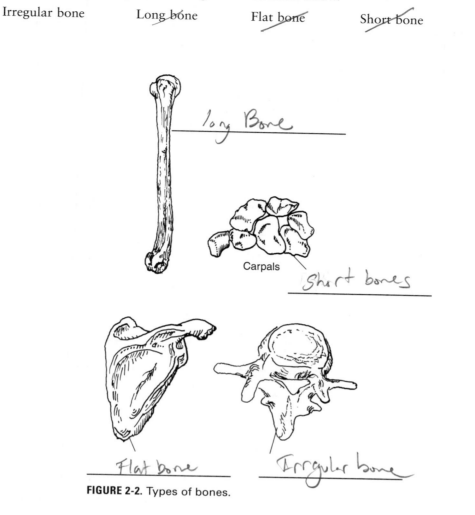

Carpals

long Bone

Short bones

Flat bone   *Irregular bone*

FIGURE 2-2. Types of bones.

■ ■ ■ **Lab Activities**

Student's Name _____ Date Due _____

1. On a skeleton, identify the bones and bone groups that make up the axial skeleton and the appendicular skeleton. List the bones that are found in each.

Skeleton	Bones and Bone Groups (i.e., carpals, ribs)
Axial	
Appendicular	

2. Using skeletons and models, find examples of the following bony landmarks. Describe where the landmark is found using terms such as proximal/distal, medial/lateral, superior/inferior, anterior/posterior and give the name of the bone where you found the landmark. Example: Trochanter: Proximal and lateral on femur.

Landmark	Location
Foramen	
Fossa	
Groove	
Meatus	
Sinus	
Condyle	
Eminence	
Facet	
Head	
Crest	
Epicondyle	
Line	
Spine	
Tubercle	
Tuberosity	
Trochanter	

3. Using the skeleton and models:
   A. Find examples of the following types of bones.
   B. Name an example of each type of bone.

Type of Bone	Example
Short	
Flat	
Long	
Irregular	
Sesamoid	

4. Using bones in the bone box, arrange the bones of the upper extremity and the bones of the lower extremity in proper anatomical orientation to one another to create the appendicular skeleton. Arrange an entire right side or left side.

■ ■ ■ **Post-Lab Questions**

Student's Name _____ Date Due _____

After you have completed the Worksheets and Lab Activities, answer the following questions without using your book or notes. When finished, check your answers.

1. Describe the following:
   A. Axial skeleton:
   Upright part of Body, head, vertebra column, Pelvis, 80 bones

   B. Appendicular skeleton:
   UE/LE, attaches to Axial Skeleton, 126 bones

2. What is bone composed of?
   _____
   _____

3. Why is cancellous bone lighter than compact bone?
   _____
   _____

4. Describe:
   A. Pressure epiphysis:
   end of long Bones, receives pressure from opposing bones making up the joint

   B. Traction epiphysis: _pulling Forces, where the tendons attach and create pulling forces_

5. What is the function of the following parts of a bone?

Bone Part	Function
Epiphysis	End of Bones, Joints/movement
Epiphyseal plate	Growth plate, of bone lengthening
Diaphysis	Great Strength, long shaft.
Medullary canal	Hollow, Decrease weight of Bone, Contains Marrow
Endosteum	Membrane lining medullary cavity - assists in Reabsorption
Osteoclasts	Bone reabsorption
Metaphysis	Supports epiphysis
Periosteum	provides nourishment, promotes growth

Articular System

Student's Name _____ Date Due _____
Complete the following questions prior to the lab class.

1. What are the three basic types of joints?
   A. _Fibrous Joints_____
   B. _Cartilaginous Joint (~~~~ Joint)_____
   C. _Synovial Joint (~~~~~~~~ ~~~)_____

2. The types of joints listed in question 3 represent which of the three basic types of joints?
   _____

3. On the following table, indicate the type of joint for each of the structures listed.

Structure	Gomphosis	Synarthrosis	Syndesmosis
Socket			
Suture			
Ligamentous			

4. Which of the previously named fibrous joints permits a slight amount of movement?
   _____

5. Give an example of each of the following types of fibrous joints.
   A. Synarthrosis
   _____ _Joint of skull_____
   B. Syndesmosis
   _____ _Distal tibiofibular Joint_____
   C. Gomphosis
   _____ _Tooth & wall of Dental socket_____

6. What is another name for a synovial joint?

_____

7. Which of the three basic types of joints provides for:

A. Mobility _____ *Synovial* _____

B. Stability _____ *Fibrous* _____

8. List an example of each of the following synovial joints:

A. Nonaxial joint _____ *Intercarpals* _____

B. Uniaxial joint _____ *Elbow* _____

C. Biaxial joint _____ *Wrist* _____

D. Triaxial joint _____ *Shoulder* _____

9. Match the following descriptions of parts of a synovial joint with the correct term. Use each term only once.

_*F*_ Enclosed cavity filled with fluid that prevents friction on moving parts.

_*D*_ Strong cord of connective tissue that attaches a muscle to another part.

_*B*_ The inside lining of the joint capsule.

_*H*_ Strong, fibrous connective tissue band that attaches bone to bone.

_*G*_ Flat, thin, fibrous sheet of connective tissue that attaches a muscle to another part.

_*A*_ Fibrous connective tissue that surrounds a joint.

_*I*_ Sheath of connective tissue that surrounds a muscle.

_*C*_ Fluid secreted from inside the lining of the joint capsule that lubricates the joint.

_*E*_ Smooth covering of bone ends.

A. Joint capsule

B. Synovial membrane

C. Synovial fluid

D. Tendon

E. Articular cartilage

F. Bursa

G. Aponeurosis

H. Ligament

I. Fascia

10. Label the drawing of a synovial joint using the following terms (Fig. 3-1):

Ligament   Joint space   Synovial membrane   Joint capsule
Bone   Synovial fluid   Articular cartilage

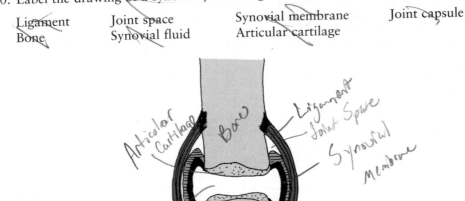

FIGURE 3-1. Synovial joint.

11. Match the following terms of pathological conditions with their definitions.

A. Fracture   _H_ Inflammation of a bursae

B. Dislocation   _D_ Injury to a ligament

C. Subluxation   _B_ Displacement of a bone from its position within a joint

D. Sprain   _A_ Disruption in the continuity of a bone

E. Tendonitis   _I_ Inflammation of a joint capsule

F. Tenosynovitis   _C_ A partial or incomplete dislocation

G. Synovitis   _J_ Injury to a muscle

H. Bursitis   _F_ Inflammation of the tendon sheath

I. Capsulitis   _E_ Inflammation of a tendon

J. Strain   _G_ Inflammation of the synovial membrane

12. Below each drawing (Figs. 3-2 through 3-4), fill in the blanks regarding planes and axes.

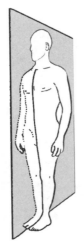

FIGURE 3-2.

A. This is the _____ plane. It is associated with the _____ axis.

Describe the direction of the axis: _____.

List the motions that occur in this plane around this axis: _____.

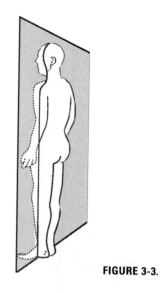

FIGURE 3-3.

B. This is the _____ plane. It is associated with the _____ axis.

Describe the direction of the axis: _____.

List the motions that occur in this plane around this axis: _____.

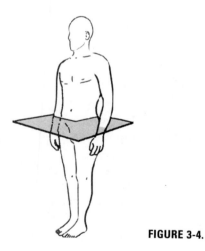

FIGURE 3-4.

C. This is the _____ plane. It is associated with the _____ axis.

Describe the direction of the axis: _____.

List the motions that occur in this plane around this axis: _____.

13. For each of the following joints, indicate the degrees of freedom for that joint.

Joint	One	Two	Three
Shoulder			
Elbow			
Wrist			
Hip			
Knee			
Ankle			

■ ■ ■ Lab Activities

Student's Name _____ Date Due _____

1. In a group, students perform as active motion the following motions.

Shoulder girdle	Elevation	Depression
	Protraction	Retraction
Shoulder	Flexion	Extension
		Hyperextension
	Abduction	Adduction
	Horizontal abduction	Horizontal adduction
	Medial rotation	Lateral rotation
Elbow	Flexion	Extension
Forearm	Supination	Pronation
Wrist	Flexion	Extension
	Radial deviation	Ulnar deviation
Thumb	Flexion	Extension
	Abduction	Opposition
Hip	Flexion	Extension
		Hyperextension
	Abduction	Adduction
	Medial rotation	Lateral rotation
Knee	Flexion	Extension
	Medial rotation	Lateral rotation
Ankle	Dorsiflexion	Plantarflexion
Foot	Inversion	Eversion

2. Using models, identify the components of synovial joints, and the location of each.

Bones	Ligaments	Capsule
Hyaline cartilage	Articular cartilage	Synovial membrane
Menisci	Labrum	Disks

3. Using models of joints or a skeleton, move the joints through the motions normally permitted to determine the degrees of freedom and the specific motions. Record your findings on the following chart.

Joint	Degrees of Freedom	Motions
Shoulder		
Elbow		
Wrist		
Hip		
Knee		

4. A. Standing next to a wall so that your left shoulder and hip are against the wall, perform flexion and extension of each of the following left side joints individually: shoulder, elbow, hip, and knee.

   In what plane were you moving? _____

   What is the axis for that plane? _____

   B. Standing with your back against a wall, your arm straight and against the wall, move your hand toward the ceiling. Still standing with your back against the wall, move your leg to the side, sliding your heel on the wall.

   What motion did you perform? _____

   In what plane were you moving? _____

   What is the axis for that plane? _____

   C. Standing facing a counter, keeping your upper arm close to your body, your elbow at 90° of flexion, and forearm pronated; move your palm along the surface of the counter.

   What motion(s) did you perform? _____

   In what plane were you moving? _____

   What is the axis for that plane? _____

   D. Sitting on a table with knee facing forward, move lower leg from side to side.

   What motion(s) did you perform? _____

   In what plane were you moving? _____

   What is the axis for that plane? _____

■ ■ ■ Post-Lab Questions

Student's Name ————————————————— Date Due ——————————

After you have completed the Worksheets and Lab Activities, answer the following questions without using your book or notes. When finished, check your answers.

1. Diarthrodial joints can be classified based on their characteristics. Fill in the blanks with the appropriate information. There may be more than one example.

Number of Axes	Shape of Joint	Joint Motions Allowed	Example
			Shoulder
		Rotation	
		Flexion/Extension	
	Condyloid		
	Saddle		
			Intercarpal

2. Check which motions generally occur in each plane about the axis of motion:

Planes/Axes	Flexion/Extension	Adduction/Abduction	Medial/Lateral Rotation
Sagittal plane Frontal axis			
Frontal plane Sagittal axis			
Transverse plane Vertical axis			

3. For the joints listed, indicate in which planes the joint normally can actively move.

Plane	Shoulder	Wrist	Knee	Ankle
Sagittal				
Frontal				
Transverse				

4. Define degrees of freedom.

_____

_____

5. Give examples of joints that have:
   A. One degree of freedom:

   _____

   _____

   B. Two degrees of freedom:

   _____

   _____

   C. Three degrees of freedom:

   _____

   _____

6. Compare and contrast fibrous joints, cartilaginous joints, and synovial joints.
   A. Compare the similarities:

   _____

   _____

   B. Contrast the differences:

   _____

   _____

7. What structure(s) may reinforce a joint capsule?

   _____

8. List the structure(s) that lubricate and supply nutrition to joint surfaces?

   _____Synovial membrane & fluid_____

9. What is the distinction between sprains and strains?

   _____Sprains injury to ligaments_____

   _____Strains - injury to muscle_____

10. List the five features of a synovial joint.

    _____

    _____

Arthrokinematics

■ ■ ■ Worksheets

Student's Name _____ Date Due _____

Complete the following questions prior to the lab class.

1. Match the following terms with their definitions.

   A. End feels   _C_ Joint motion

   B. Arthrokinematic motion   _F_ Forceful external force within a short range

   C. Osteokinematic motion   _E_ Slow passive external force

   D. Joint play   _B_ Joint surface motion

   E. Joint mobilization   _D_ Accessory joint movement produced by an external force

   F. Manipulation   _A_ Nature of the resistance at the end of joint range

2. Match the types of end feels with their definitions.

   A. Bony end feel   _C_ No mechanical limitation

   B. Capsular end feel   _A_ Hard and abrupt limit

   C. Empty end feel   _B_ Leatherlike with slight give

3. Match the terms for arthrokinematic motion with their definitions.

   A. Roll   _B_ Same point on each surface remains in contact with each other

   B. Spin   _C_ One point on a joint surface contacts new points on the other surface

   C. Glide   _A_ New points on each surface come into contact throughout the motion

4. Match the joint surface position with its description.

   A. Congruent joint surfaces   _A_ Close-packed position

   B. Incongruent joint surfaces   _B_ Loose-packed position

5. Match the type of force with its definition.

   A. Traction, distraction or tension force   _A_ Joint surfaces are pulled apart

   B. Approximation, compression force   _C_ Joint surfaces move parallel and in opposite directions of each other

   C. Shear force   _B_ Joint surfaces are pushed closer together

6. Give one example of each of the following:
   A. Springy block:

   _____

   _____

   B. Soft tissue approximation:

   _____

   _____

   C. Muscle guarding:

   _____

   _____

7. Apply the concave-convex rule to identify the surface moving in each of the following statements.

   The ____Convex____ joint surfaces move in the opposite direction of the joint movement.

   The ____Concave____ joint surfaces move in the same direction as the joint motion.

■ ■ ■ Lab Activities

Student's Name _____ Date Due _____

1. Perform the following on several people. Describe the end feel of each motion.

Motion	End Feel
Elbow flexion	
Elbow extension	
Wrist flexion	
Knee extension	
Hip flexion with knee flexion	
Hip flexion with knee extended	

2. Perform shoulder flexion first while maintaining medial rotation and then with lateral rotation. Compare the amount of range of motion achieved with each movement.
   A. Which movement has greater ROM?

   _____ medial rotation   _____ lateral rotation

   B. This is an example of what type of arthrokinematics motion?

   _____

3. Sitting, facing your partner with your partner's hand supported on a table, grasp your partner's middle phalange of his or her index finger with one hand and the distal phalange of your partner's index finger with your other hand. While holding the middle phalange stable, move the distal phalange side to side.

A. Is this a movement that a person can voluntary perform?

_____

B. What is this movement called?

_____

4. Using a skeleton and bones locate bones whose articular surfaces have the following characteristics. Name the bone and describe where on the bone the characteristic is found (proximal/distal; medial/lateral; anterior/posterior).

A. Concave surface

Bone	Location
Ulna	Proximal
Tibia	Proximal
Phalanx	Proximal
Glenoid Fossa	lateral / Posterior
Acetabulum	lateral

B. Convex surface

Bone	Location
Femur	Distal
Metacarpal	Distal
Humerus	Proximal / Medial
Femur	Medial
Tibia	Distal / Anterior

C. Examine the carpometacarpal (CMC) joint of the thumb and fingers.

1) How are the joint surfaces of the thumb different from the joint surfaces of the fingers?

Fingers are two motion surfaces, But
the thumb is more convex creating more
movement

2) What is the type of joint for each?

Modified Uniaxial

5. Observe the distal end of a femur and the proximal end of a tibia.

   A. Which has the larger articular surface?

   _____ Femur _____

   B. Move the tibia on the femur as if performing extension and flexion. Does the tibia move over the entire articular surface of the femur?

   _____ No _____

   C. As you move the tibia on the femur as if performing extension, move the femur posteriorly on the tibia. Did the tibia move over more of the articular surface of the femur this time?

   _____ Yes _____

   The posterior movement of the femur is an example of what kind of arthrokinematic motion?

   _____ Joint Play _____

6. Using a skeleton or articulated upper extremity bones, observe the proximal end of the radius as pronation and supination are performed.

   A. Describe the movement of the radius on the humerus.

   _____

   _____

   B. This movement is an example of what type of arthrokinematic motion?

   _____

7. Using a skeleton or articulated upper extremity bones, observe the movement of the head of the humerus as shoulder joint medial and lateral rotation are performed. Indicate which of the following movements occurs as the humerus moves on the glenoid fossa.

   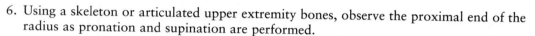

   _____ Roll   _____ Spin   _____ Glide

8. Place two small sticky notes with large dots on the lateral surface of your partner's arm with one dot over the lateral epicondyle at the elbow and the other at the shoulder on the greater tubercle. As your partner slowly flexes the shoulder observe the positions of the dots.

   A. When performing shoulder flexion, which joint surface is moving the concave or the convex surface?

   _____

   B. In the starting position the dot at the elbow is _____ to the dot at the shoulder.

   C. At the end of shoulder flexion the dot at the elbow is _____ to the dot at the shoulder.

   D. This is an example of the concave-convex rule describing movement of the convex joint surface. According to the concave-convex rule, the convex joint surface moves in

   the _____ direction as the body segment's motion.

9. Place two small sticky notes with large dots on the lateral aspect of your partner's lower leg with one dot over the lateral malleolus and the other over the head of the fibula. Observe the positions of the dots as your partner performs knee flexion moving the tibia on the femur.

   A. When performing knee flexion and extension moving the tibia on the femur, which joint surface is moving—the concave or the convex surface?

   _____

   B. In what direction did the proximal dot move?

   _____

   C. In what direction did the distal dot move?

   _____

   D. This is an example of the concave-convex rule describing movement of the concave joint surface. According to the concave-convex rule, the concave joint surface moves

   in the _____ direction as the body segment's motion.

10. Using a skeleton or bones, observe the close-packed or open-packed positions of the following joints.

Joint	Close-Packed	Open-Packed
Glenohumeral	Abduction and lateral rotation	55° abduction, 30° horizontal adduction
Elbow: ulnohumeral	Extension	70° flexion, 10° supination
Interphalangeal	Full extension	Slight flexion
Hip	Full extension and medial rotation	30° flexion, 30° abduction and slight lateral rotation
Knee	Full extension and lateral rotation of tibia	25° flexion
Ankle: talocrural	Full dorsiflexion	10° plantar flexion, midway between inversion and eversion

11. Describe, and if possible perform, typical exercises or activities that apply

   A. A traction force through the upper extremities.

   _____

   _____

   B. An approximation force through the lower extremities.

   _____

   _____

12. Using an articulated model of the spine, bend the column of vertebra to the left.
    A. On which side are structures compressed?

    _____

    B. On which side are structures under tension?

    _____

    C. Straighten the vertebral column and twist the column to the right. What force is being applied to the structures?

    _____

■ ■ ■ Post-Lab Questions

Student's Name _____ Date Due _____

After you have completed the Worksheets and Lab Activities, answer the following questions without using your book or notes. When finished, check your answers.

1. Give an example of each of the following, try to use examples not in the textbook.

    A. Bony end feel:

    _____

    B. Capsular end feel:

    _____

    C. Soft tissue approximation:

    _____

    D. Joint movement with large amount of roll:

    _____

    E. Joint movement with large amount of glide:

    _____

    F. Joint movement with large amount of spin:

    _____

2. When a person assumes sitting from standing, the knee is flexing.
    A. When performing this movement, is the concave surface moving on the convex surface or is the convex surface moving on the concave surface? Underline the correct response.
    B. Based on this example, according to the concave-convex law, when the _Convex_ surface moves on the _Concave_ surface, the _Convex_ joint surface moves in the _opposite_ direction as the body segment movement.
3. Is accessory motion or joint play possible in a close-packed or an open-packed position? Why?
    open-packed _position_ _because_ _the_ _joint_
    _is_ _not_ _compressed._

Muscular System

Student's Name _____ Date Due _____

Complete the following questions prior to the lab class.

1. Match the following terms with their definition.

   A. Reversal of muscle action   _____ Muscle contraction without joint movement

   B. Normal resting length   _____ Can produce hand opening and closing

   C. Tone   _____ The origin of the contracting muscle moves
                                                 toward the insertion

   D. Tenodesis   _____ Constant speed variable resistance

   E. Isometric contraction   _____ Not as powerful as the prime mover

   F. Isokinetic contraction   _____ Slight tension in a muscle

   G. Assisting mover   _____ Position when muscle is unstimulated

2. Muscles have origins and insertions. Which is generally proximal?

   A. Origin   B. Insertion

3. Using the following terms, identify the muscle shapes illustrated in Figure 5-1.

   Triangular   Strap   Rhomboidal   Fusiform
   Bipennate   Multipennate   Unipennate

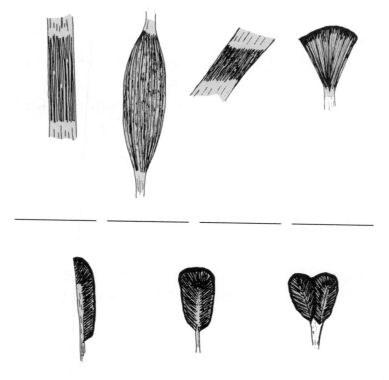

_____ _____ _____ _____

_____ _____ _____   **FIGURE 5-1.** Muscle shapes.

4. Match the muscle characteristic with the correct description. Use each term once.

   A. Irritability   _____ Ability to be stretched beyond normal resting length

   B. Contractility   _____ Ability to receive and respond to a stimulus

   C. Extensibility   _____ Ability to produce tension

   D. Elasticity   _____ Ability to return to normal length

5. Identify the type of muscle contraction described as being eccentric (E) or concentric (C).

   _____ Lengthening contraction

   _____ Shortening contraction

   _____ Insertion moves toward origin

   _____ Insertion moves away from origin

   _____ Isotonic contraction

   _____ Muscle contraction moves the body segment against gravity

   _____ Muscle contraction slows the pull of gravity on the body segment

6. Complete the following statements using the terms listed to fill in the blanks.

   Agonist   Antagonist   Cocontraction   Neutralizer   Stabilizer   Synergist

   A. The shoulder girdle muscles act as _____ when one lifts a book off the table.

   B. When a muscle acts to eliminate undesired motions during an activity, the muscle is functioning as a _____.

   C. Contracting the quadriceps and hamstrings muscles simultaneously is an example of

   _____.

   D. Muscles that are primarily responsible for producing a specific movement are called

   _____.

   E. When the biceps are contracting the triceps muscle is the _____.

   F. The elbow has three muscles that can produce flexion. When more than one is working, the muscles are acting as the _____.

   G. When the wrist flexors and extensors produce ulnar deviation, each muscle is also acting as a _____.

7. A muscle that shortens approximately 2 inches and can be lengthened 4 inches has an

   _____ of how many inches? _____

8. For each of the following activities, indicate if it is an example of an open kinetic chain or a closed kinetic chain.

   _____ A. The upper extremity when one is walking carrying a book bag

   _____ B. The upper extremity when one is doing push-ups

   _____ C. The upper extremity when one is supported on crutches

   _____ D. The lower extremities when one is swinging from an overhead bar

   _____ E. The lower extremities when one is performing wall slides

   _____ F. The lower extremity being used to kick a ball

9. A muscle that cannot be lengthened simultaneously over all the joints it crosses is said to be: (Select the correct answer.)

   _____ Actively insufficient   _____ Passively insufficient

Muscle Strength Grades

There are a number of methods used to test the torque-generating capabilities of muscles (commonly called muscle strength). Manual muscle testing is a well-documented method used to evaluate muscle strength. Two methods of grading are commonly used to report strength testing results. One method uses numbers 0–5 and the other uses letters. For better distinction between grades, some also used + and − with the number or letter grade. Based on the definitions of muscle-testing grades, a person is placed in different positions when determining different muscle grades. Laboratory activities in this manual directing the student to palpate muscle origin, insertion, and belly, are designed to be carried out in the muscle-testing position for a grade of Fair, F, or 3. This means that these palpations are performed in a position that requires the muscle to contract against the resistance of gravity.

Definition	Letter Grade	Number Grade
The absence of muscle contraction.	0; zero	0/5
The ability to produce a muscle contraction that is detectable by palpation or observation, but is not strong enough to cause joint movement.	T; trace	1/5
The ability to produce a muscle contraction that causes complete joint motion without the resistance of gravity.	P; poor	2/5
The ability to produce a muscle contraction that causes complete joint motion against the resistance of gravity.	F; fair	3/5
The ability to produce a muscle contraction that causes complete joint motion against gravity and withstands moderate manual resistance to an isometric contraction but yields against maximal manual resistance.	G; good	4/5
The ability to produce a muscle contraction that causes complete joint motion against gravity and withstands maximal resistance to an isometric contraction.	N; normal	5/5

■ ■ ■ Lab Activities

Student's Name _____ Date Due _____

1. Palpate the origins and insertions of the following muscles. Indicate which, origin or insertion, is located proximally and which is located distally.

Muscle	Origin	Insertion	Proximal	Distal
Brachioradialis	Lateral supracondylar ridge on the humerus	Styloid process of the radius	Origin	Insertion
Teres minor	Axillary border of scapula	Greater tubercle of humerus		
Rectus abdominis	Pubis	Costal cartilages of 5th, 6th, & 7th ribs		
Sartorius	Anterior superior iliac spine	Proximal medial aspect of tibia		
Soleus	Posterior tibia and fibula	Posterior calcaneous		

2. Locate pictures of the following muscles and then locate the muscle on your partner and yourself.

   A. Using a skin pencil or water soluble markers draw over the muscle showing the muscle fiber arrangement.

   B. Indicate the name for the type of muscle fiber arrangement for each muscle using the following terms:

Parallel	Oblique	Strap	Fusiform	Rhomboidal
Unipennate	Bipennate	Multipennate	Triangular	

Muscle	Fiber Arrangement
Deltoid	
Pectoralis major	
Flexor pollicis longus	
Biceps brachii	
Rectus femoris	
Sternocleidomastoid	
Rhomboids	

3. Have your partner assume a supine position. Standing next to your partner's right lower extremity, place the heel of his or her right lower extremity in the palm of your right hand. Place your left hand under your partner's right thigh. Slowly flex, and then extend, your partner's hip and knee simultaneously. Note the amount of "resistance" you feel to your moving your partner's lower extremity. Some people have a difficult time letting someone else move their body parts, however, if your partner is relaxed, you are feeling the normal resting tone of your partner's lower extremity muscles.

4. With your partner in a supine position. Standing next to your partner's right lower extremity, place the heel of his or her right lower extremity in the palm of your right hand. Place your left hand under your partner's right thigh. Slowly flex, and then extend, your partner's hip and knee simultaneously. Note the amount of hip flexion. Next, slowly flex, and then extend, your partner's hip while keeping the knee extended (straight). Note the amount of hip flexion your partner has when the knee remains extended. Hip flexion with the knee extended (straight) is known as a straight leg raise—SLR.

   A. Was the amount of hip flexion more, the same, or less with knee extended compared to hip flexion with the knee flexed? _____

   B. Was the result what you expected? _____

   C. Is this an example of active or passive insufficiency? _____

   D. Which muscle(s) was (were) being lengthened simultaneously over all the joints they cross when you moved your partner through the SLR?

   _____

5. With your partner in a supine position, again perform simultaneous hip and knee flexion. Note the amount of knee flexion obtained when the hip is flexed. Have your partner assume a prone position. Align the thigh in anatomical position. Slowly flex the knee of the same lower extremity you had moved when your partner was in supine. Note the amount of knee flexion motion present now that the hip is extended.

   A. Was the amount of knee flexion more, the same, or less with the hip extended

   compared to knee flexion with the hip flexed? _____

   B. Was the result what you expected? _____

   C. Is this an example of active or passive insufficiency? _____

   D. Which muscle(s) was (were) being lengthened simultaneously over all the joints they

   cross when you moved your partner through the SLR? _____

6. A. With your partner sitting over the side of a treatment table with his or her knee at about 90° of flexion, resist your partner's isometric knee flexion. Note how strong the knee flexors are in this position.

   B. Have your partner assume a prone position with hip extended and the same knee flexed to 90°. Repeat the resisted isometric contraction of the knee flexors noting the strength of the knee flexors.

   C. Have your partner assume a prone position with hip extended, flex his or her knee through as much of its range of motion as possible (more than 90°). Repeat the resisted isometric contraction at the end of the motion noting the strength of the knee flexors. Be cautious with the resistance offered because your partner may develop a muscle cramp.

   Describe the hip and knee position in these three scenarios:

Hip and Knee Position	Hip	Knee
A. Sitting on side of table		
B. Prone with knee at 90°		
C. Prone with maximum knee flexion		

   D. Was the strength of the knee flexors the same in all three positions? _____

   E. If not, in which position were the knee flexors:

   Stronger? _____ Weaker? _____

   F. Is this an example of active or passive insufficiency? _____

7. In the prone position when your partner performs the maximum knee flexion he or she can, how do you determine if he or she is experiencing active insufficiency of the knee flexors or passive insufficiency of the knee extensors?

   _____

   _____

8. Throughout this lab manual you will be asked to analyze activities to determine the type of muscle contractions required to perform the activity. The general rule is: when a muscle is acting to *overcome* gravity or body weight, the muscle is performing a concentric (shortening) contraction and when a muscle is acting to *slow down* gravity, the muscle is performing an eccentric (lengthening) contraction.

In the supine position perform a straight leg raise.

A. Name the muscle group acting at the hip to perform the SLR. _____

B. Name the antagonist muscle group at the hip. _____

C. As the leg is raised, select the type of contraction the hip agonist is performing:

_____ Isometric   _____ Concentric   _____ Eccentric   _____ None

D. As the leg is lowered, select the type of contraction the hip agonist is performing:

_____ Isometric   _____ Concentric   _____ Eccentric   _____ None

E. As the leg is raised, select the type of contraction the hip antagonist is performing:

_____ Isometric   _____ Concentric   _____ Eccentric   _____ None

F. As the leg is lowered, select the type of contraction the hip antagonist is performing:

_____ Isometric   _____ Concentric   _____ Eccentric   _____ None

G. Name the muscle group acting at the knee to maintain it extended. _____

H. Name the antagonist muscle group at the knee. _____

I. As the leg is raised, select the type of contraction the knee agonist is performing:

_____ Isometric   _____ Concentric   _____ Eccentric   _____ None

J. As the leg is lowered, select the type of contraction the knee agonist is performing:

_____ Isometric   _____ Concentric   _____ Eccentric   _____ None

K. As the leg is raised, select the type of contraction the knee antagonist is performing:

_____ Isometric   _____ Concentric   _____ Eccentric   _____ None

L. As the leg is lowered, select the type of contraction the knee antagonist is performing:

_____ Isometric   _____ Concentric   _____ Eccentric   _____ None

M. When joint movement occurs against gravity, the agonist performs which type of contraction?

_____ Isometric   _____ Concentric   _____ Eccentric   _____ None

N. When joint movement occurs against gravity, the antagonist performs which type of contraction?

_____ Isometric   _____ Concentric   _____ Eccentric   _____ None

O. When a joint is moved against gravity by action of another joint, to prevent movement the agonist performs which type of contraction?

_____ Isometric   _____ Concentric   _____ Eccentric   _____ None

P. When joint movement occurs in the same direction that gravity would produce movement, the agonist performs which type of contraction?

_____ Isometric   _____ Concentric   _____ Eccentric   _____ None

Q. When performing an eccentric contraction, the agonist is acting to (select one):

_____ Overcome gravity   _____ Slow down gravity

R. When performing a concentric contraction, the agonist is acting to (select one):

_____ Overcome gravity   _____ Slow down gravity

9. Examining the location of the biceps brachii on the anterior surface of the arm, the insertion of its tendon on the radius indicates that the biceps will flex the elbow and supinate the forearm.

A. When the elbow is in extension with forearm supination and the biceps performs an isometric contraction, because of the angle of pull what force does the biceps exert on the elbow?

———— Approximation　　　　　———— Traction

B. When the elbow is in full flexion with forearm supination and the biceps performs an isometric contraction, because of the angle of pull, what force does the biceps exert on the elbow?

———— Approximation　　　　　———— Traction

10. Move from a sitting to a standing position.

A. The lower extremities are moving in:

———— An open kinetic chain　　　　———— A closed kinetic chain

B. Which hip and knee muscle groups are the agonists?

———— Extensors　　　　　　———— Flexors

C. The agonists perform:

———— Concentric contractions　　　———— Eccentric contractions

———— Isometric contractions　　　———— No contraction

11. From a standing position, sit down.

A. The lower extremities are moving in:

———— An open kinetic chain　　　　———— A closed kinetic chain

B. Which muscle groups are the agonists?

———— Extensors　　　　　　———— Flexors

C. The agonists perform:

———— Concentric contractions　　　———— Eccentric contractions

———— Isometric contractions　　　———— No contraction

■ ■ ■ Post-Lab Questions

Student's Name ————————————————————— Date Due —————————————

After you have completed the Worksheets and Lab Activities, answer the following questions without using your book or notes. When finished, check your answers.

1. When the agonist is contracting to overcome the resistance of gravity, the body part is moving in the opposite direction as the force of gravity. The type of contraction the agonist is performing is:

———— Concentric　　　———— Eccentric　　　————Isometric

2. When the agonist is contracting to slow down the force of gravity, the body part is moving in the:

_____ Same direction as the force of gravity

_____ Opposite direction as the force of gravity

The agonist is contracting

_____ Concentrically   _____ Eccentrically   _____ Isometrically

3. When the agonist is contracting isotonically, the antagonist is _____

4. A. In sitting, you raise your arm through full range of motion. The agonists are the shoulder:

_____ Flexors   _____ Extensors

B. In sitting, you lower your arm to the anatomical position from full flexion. The agonists are the shoulder:

_____ Flexors   _____ Extensors

C. In supine, you raise your arm through full ROM. The agonists are:

_____

_____

D. In supine, you return your arm to the anatomical position from full flexion. The agonists are:

_____

_____

5. If the elbow joint was designed to have abduction ROM under voluntary control, what would be the location of the muscle(s) that would perform elbow abduction.

_____

_____

6. In the sitting position with the upper extremity in the anatomical position, curl (flex) just your fingers as much as possible. Now flex your wrist. Which of the following may be true?

_____ A. Passive insufficiency of the finger flexors

_____ B. Passive insufficiency of the finger extensors

_____ C. Passive insufficiency of the wrist flexors

_____ D. Passive insufficiency of the wrist extensors

_____ E. Active insufficiency of the finger flexors

_____ F. Active insufficiency of the finger extensors

_____ G. Active insufficiency of the wrist flexors

_____ H. Active insufficiency of the wrist extensors

The Nervous System

■ ■ ■ Worksheets

Student's Name _____ Date Due _____

Complete the following questions prior to the lab class.

1. Match the following terms and descriptors.

   A. Neurons

   B. Cell body

   C. Myelin

   D. Neurilemma

   E. Nerve fiber

   F. Tract

   G. Anterior root (ventral)

   H. Posterior root (dorsal)

   I. Interneuron

   J. Cerebrum

   K. Cerebral hemispheres

   L. Corpus callosum

   M. Cortex

   N. Upper motor neurons

   O. Lower motor neurons

   _____ Synapse occurs above (proximal) to the anterior horn

   _____ Nerve cell

   _____ Holds sensory neuron

   _____ Conductor of impulses for neuron

   _____ Transparent tissue around myelin

   _____ Joins the cerebral hemispheres

   _____ Deals with highest mental functions

   _____ White fatty tissue around the PNS and CNS

   _____ Holds motor neurons

   _____ Outer coating of brain

   _____ Transmits sensory, motor, or both, impulses

   _____ Synapse occurs below (distal) to the anterior horn

   _____ Bundle of nerve fibers

   _____ Contains the nucleus

   _____ There are two of these

2. Complete the following table.

Lobe	Location in Brain	Main Function
Frontal		
Occipital		
Parietal		
Temporal		

3. Match each of the following structures with its major function.

_B_ Thalamus   A. Hormone function and behavior

_A_ Hypothalamus   B. Body sensations—where pain is perceived

_D_ Basal ganglia   C. Automatic control of respiration

_F_ Midbrain   D. Coordination of motor movement

_C_ Medulla oblongata   E. Control of muscle coordination, tone, posture

_E_ Cerebellum   F. Coordination of visual reflexes

4. Match the spinal cord coverings with their location.

A. Arachnoid mater   _____ Outer layer

B. Dura mater   _____ Middle layer

C. Pia mater   _____ Inner layer

5. The subarachnoid space is located between the _____ and the _____ spinal cord coverings. What circulates through this space?

_____

6. Match the arteries with the areas they supply.

A. External carotid arteries   _____ Arterial system supplying blood to brain

B. Internal carotid arteries   _____ Supplies the occipital lobes

C. Basilar artery   _____ Joins the anterior and posterior cerebral arteries

D. Posterior cerebral arteries   _____ Supplies the cerebellum, pons, and midbrain

E. Circle of Willis   _____ Joins the right and left cerebral arteries

F. Posterior communicating artery   _____ Supplies the scalp, dura, and skull

G. Anterior communicating artery   _____ Supplies the anterior part of the brain

7. Match the following spinal cord elements with their descriptions.

A. Conus medullaris   _____ Contains neuronal cell bodies

B. Cauda equine   _____ End of spinal cord

C. Filum terminale   _____ Collection of nerve roots

D. Gray matter   _____ Non-neural portion of spinal cord

8. What is the function of cerebral spinal fluid?

_____

9. Label the drawing of a vertebra using the terms given (Fig. 6-1):

Vertebral foramen   Body   Neural arch

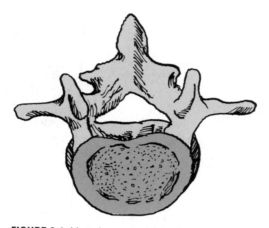

FIGURE 6-1. Vertebra, superior view.

10. Label the cross section drawing of the spinal cord using the terms given (Fig. 6-2):

| Gray matter | Posterior horn | Anterior horn | Peripheral nerve |
| Posterior columns | White matter | Posterior root | Anterior root |

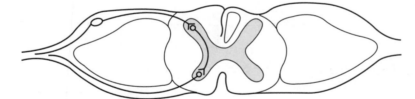

FIGURE 6-2. Spinal cord.

11. Match the cranial nerve name with the cranial nerve number.

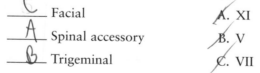

_C_ Facial   A. XI

_A_ Spinal accessory   B. V

_B_ Trigeminal   C. VII

12. How many pairs of spinal nerve are there? How many in each section of the vertebral column?

Cervical _____   Thoracic _____   Lumbar _____

Sacral _____   Coccygeal _____

13. Indicate whether the following spinal nerves exit above or below the vertebra of the same number. If there is not a matching vertebra, indicate which vertebra it exits below.

Nerve	Above	Below	Vertebra
C1			
C7			
C8			
T1			

14. The spinal nerve divides into the posterior (dorsal) ramus and the anterior (ventral) ramus. What is the function of each ramus?

    Posterior (dorsal) ramus _____

    Anterior (ventral) ramus) _____

15. List the major muscle groups innervated by each of the following spinal segments:

    A. C1–C3 ___FAcial   Muscles / Neck_____

    B. C5–C6 _Shoulder Abductors ,   Deltoids , Biceps_____

    C. C6–T1 ___Triceps ,   Extensors ,   Elbows Ext._____
    Thumb ext.

    D. T2–T12 ___Intercostals , Serratus Anterior_____

    E. L2–L4 ___Quads , adductors, Toe extensors ,___
    knee extension   DF

    F. L4–S3 ___Hamstrings / Calves ,   Hip ext , knee ✓___
    PF

16. For each of the three major nerve plexuses provide the spinal levels that combine to make the plexus.

    A. Cervical plexus: ___C1–C3_____

    B. Brachial plexus: ___C4– T1_____

    C. Lumbar plexus: ___L1–L5_____

    Lumbar portion: _____

    Sacral portion: ___S1–S3_____

17. On the drawing of the nervous system (Fig. 6-3), identify and label the following structures:

Afferent neuron	Axon terminals	Axon
Sensory receptor	Dendrites	Myelin sheath
Efferent neuron	Node of Ranvier	

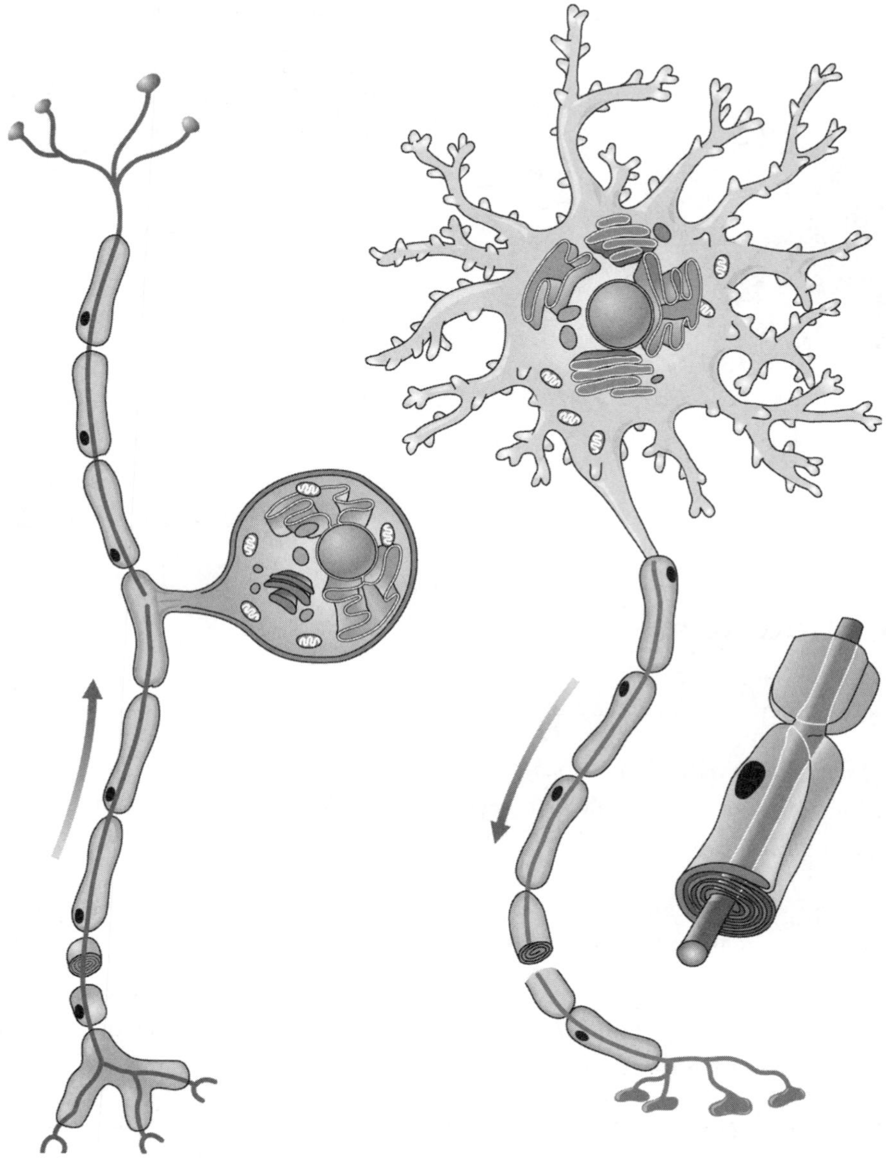

FIGURE 6-3. Neuron structure. (From Scanlon, VC, and Sanders, T: Essentials of Anatomy and Physiology, ed 4. FA Davis, Philadelphia, 2003, p 157, with permission.)

18. On the drawing of the brachial plexus (Fig. 6-4), label the following structures:

Cords   Nerve roots   Peripheral nerves   Trunks

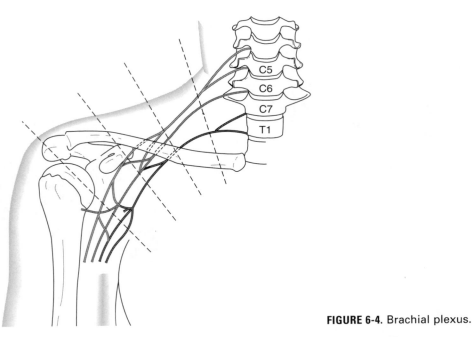

FIGURE 6-4. Brachial plexus.

■ ■ ■ Lab Activities

Student's Name _____ Date Due _____

1. Using a model of the spinal column, locate:
   A. The divisions of the vertebral column—cervical, thoracic, lumbar, sacral, and coccyx.
   B. The intervertebral foramen.

2. Place stockinet on your arm and leg, draw on the stockinet the sensory dermatomes. These stockinets can be used as study guides for reviewing sensory dermatomes.

3. Place stockinet on your arm and leg, draw on the stockinet the peripheral nerves and their sensory distribution. These stockinets can be used as study guides for reviewing peripheral nerves and their sensory distribution.

4. Compare the areas of sensory dermatomes to the areas of sensory distribution of the peripheral nerves.

5. Using models of the brain and skull, locate the lobes of the brain. Note the relationship of the lobes within the skull.

6. Using string or yarn of different colors, construct models of the brachial and lumbar plexuses.

7. Using the skeleton, arrange string or yarn to illustrate the pathways of the peripheral nerves.

8. After completing activity 7, locate those areas on your partner where peripheral nerves are close to the surface and palpate these areas. Describe what you feel as you palpate and what it feels like when your partner palpates these areas on you.

9. Describe and assume the postures resulting from the following nerve injuries. Identify the nerve involved.

Posture	Description	Nerve
Erb's palsy		
Scapular winging		
Wrist drop		
Ape hand		
Pope's blessing		
Claw hand		
Drop foot		

■ ■ ■ Post-Lab Questions

Student's Name _____ Date Due _____

After you have completed the Worksheets and Lab Activities, answer the following questions without using your book or notes. When finished, check your answers.

1. Underline the correct response in the (   ).

   Efferent information originates in the (spinal cord/periphery) and is about (sensory/motor) function. Afferent information originates in the (spinal cord/periphery) and is about (sensory/motor) function.

2. On the following table, indicate if the structures are part of the central nervous system (CNS) or the peripheral nervous system (PNS).

Structure	CNS	PNS
Median nerve		X
Brain stem	X	
Parietal lobe	X	
Anterior horn		X
Corticospinal tract	X	
Nerve roots		X
Femoral nerve		X

3. Match the following motions with the peripheral nerve that innervates the muscle(s) responsible for that motion.

___E___ Forearm pronation   A. Ulnar

___D___ Shoulder abduction   B. Radial

___B___ Elbow extension   C. Musculocutaneous

___A___ Wrist ulnar deviation   D. Axillary

___C___ Elbow flexion   E. Median

4. Match the following movements with the peripheral nerve that innervates the muscle(s) responsible for that motion.

___C___ Hip adduction   A. Peroneal

___A___ Ankle dorsiflexion   B. Sciatic

___E___ Knee extension   C. Obturator

___D___ Toe flexion   D. Tibial

___B___ Hip extension   E. Femoral

5. The brachial plexus has three trunks. Match each trunk with the spinal level(s) that supply the trunk.

___B___ Superior   A. C8–T1

___C___ Middle   B. C5–C6

___A___ Inferior   C. C7

6. Match the major nerves that supply the lower extremity with the associated spinal level.

___B___ Femoral   A. L4–S3

___A___ Sciatic   B. L2–L4

7. Match each of the following impairments with the nerve injury that may cause it.

___B___ Scapular winging   A. Ulnar nerve

___D___ Wrist drop   B. Long thoracic nerve

___C___ Ape hand   C. Median nerve

___A___ Claw hand   D. Radial nerve

8. What are the two nerves that the sciatic nerve divides into?

_____Tibial_____ / _____Common Peroneal_____

Basic Biomechanics

■ ■ ■ Worksheets

Student's Name _____ Date Due _____

Complete the following questions prior to the lab class.

1. Match the following terms with their definitions.

   _____ Mechanics   A. Study of the structure and function of the human body

   _____ Biomechanics   B. Factors associated with moving systems

   _____ Dynamics   C. Study of forces and the motions they produce

   _____ Statics   D. Factors associated with nonmoving systems

2. A. The two types of mechanical quantities are _____ and _____.

   B. Force is which type of quantity? _____

   C. Force has two types of components, which are _____ and _____.

3. A. A scalar quantity has only _____.

   B. Examples of things measured in scalar are _____, _____,

   and _____.

4. Match the following terms with their definitions.

   _____ Inertia   A. Tendency of a force to produce rotation about an axis

   _____ Torque   B. Force that tends to prevent motion of one surface across anther

   _____ Friction   C. Vector that describes speed

   _____ Velocity   D. Resistance to any change of its motion in either speed or direction

5. Gravity is the mutual attraction between the _____ and an _____.
   Gravitational force is always directed _____ to the center of the earth.

6. Describe how the mechanical advantage of a lever is determined.

   _____

7. List the two purposes for using a pulley.

   A. _____

   B. _____

8. Label each of the following examples with the appropriate law of Newton.

   Law of inertia   Law of acceleration   Law of action-reaction

   A. A person with a complete spinal cord injury at C5 is in a manual wheelchair race with a person with a complete spinal cord injury at T10. The wheelchairs and the weight of the racers are equal. Which of Newton's laws explains why the patient with a T10 level injury is likely to win?

   _____

   B. A person with weakness of the left shoulder muscles is sitting with the shoulder and elbow in the anatomical position. A weighted cuff is placed about the person's left wrist with instructions to lift the arm and weight 10 times. In addition to weakness making this a challenging exercise, which of Newton's laws explains why initiating the movement is difficult?

   _____

   C. A plyometric exercise involves tossing a weighted ball against a trampoline. When the ball is caught upon its return, rather than stopping the ball immediately one grasps the ball and moves the arms in the same direction as the ball was moving before tossing the ball again. Which of Newton's laws explains the rebound of the ball off the trampoline?

   _____

   Which of Newton's laws explains not stopping the ball immediately and moving with the ball?

   _____

9. Draw examples of linear forces, parallel forces, and concurrent forces and include the resultant force.

10. If the rower pictured (Fig. 7-1) pulls on one oar and pushes on the other what will happen?

   _____ This maneuver is an example of a _____.

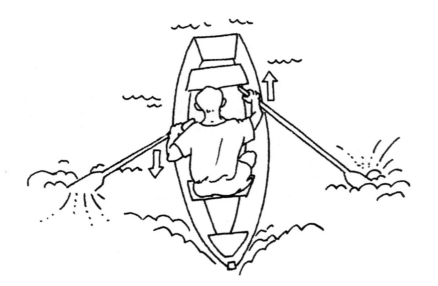

FIGURE 7-1. Rowboat.

11. Where is the center of gravity of the body considered to be located in an adult?

_____

12. In many countries women transport objects by carrying them on top of their heads. What happens to the center of gravity when an object is carried in this manner?

_____

13. A person with only one leg has a _____ base of support when standing than a person with two legs. Centering the center of gravity over the base of support when standing is achieved by postural adjustments that may contribute to musculoskeletal

    stress. Providing an ambulatory assistive device such as a walker _____ the base of support reducing the musculoskeletal stress.

14. Identify the class of lever of each of the tools below (Fig. 7-2) and indicate the axis (A), resistance (R), and the force (F).

Implement	Class of Lever
Barbecue tongs	
Pliers	
Nutcracker	

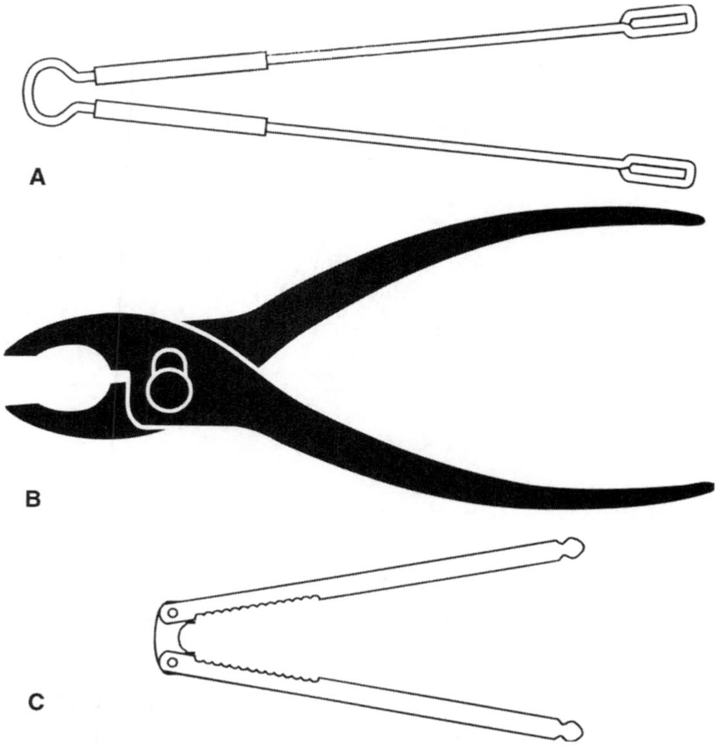

FIGURE 7-2. *(A)* Barbecue tongs, *(B)* pliers, and *(C)* nutcracker.

■ ■ ■ Lab Activities

Student's Name _____ Date Due _____

1. In a standing position, perform shoulder flexion while maintaining the elbow in extension and with a weighted cuff held in the hand. Repeat with the weighted cuff secured above the elbow.

   A. Which is easier? Why?

   _____

   B. What is the effect on the center of gravity when the shoulder is at 90° of flexion?

   _____

   C. What is the effect on the center of gravity when the shoulder is at 180° of flexion?

   _____

2. Assume the hands and knees position.

   First, lift one hand off the floor.

   Second, (replace the hand on the floor and) lift one leg off the floor.

   Third, lift one hand and the opposite leg off the floor.

   Fourth, lift the hand and leg on the same side off the floor.

   A. Which position is most stable?

   _____

   B. Which is most unstable?

   _____

   C. Explain why?

   _____

   _____

3. Standing with your back and legs against the wall, attempt to pick up an object on the floor about 5 inches in front of your toes without flexing your knees.

   A. Could you pick up the object?

   _____

   B. Explain.

   _____

4. Stand with one foot on each side of a doorjamb such that your forefoot is beyond the door frame and your nose touches the door frame. Rise up on your toes.

   A. Could you rise up on your toes?

   _____

   B. Explain.

   _____

   _____

5. With your partner behind you as a spotter:

   Sitting in a wheelchair with your feet on the footplates, wheel up a ramp.

   Repeat with a backpack full of books or weights attached to the back of the wheelchair.

   Repeat sitting tailor style (or with your feet on the seat) and the footrests removed.

   A. Compare the effort to propel up the ramp in each attempt. _____

   _____

   B. What happened when the backpack was on the back of the wheelchair?

   _____

   _____

   C. What happened when your feet were on the seat of the wheelchair?

   _____

   _____

   D. Explain.

   _____

   _____

6. Repeat the activities in question 5 using an amputee wheelchair. (If an amputee wheelchair is not available, add weighted cuffs to the footplates of a standard wheelchair.)

   A. Were the results the same as when using a standard wheelchair? _____

   _____

   B. Explain. _____

   _____

7. Given that stability depends on the relationship of the center of gravity (COG) to the base of support (BOS), what happens when you reach for objects placed to each side and in front of you while in the following positions?

   Kneeling   Heelsitting   Standing   Sitting on the side of a treatment table

   A. Describe what happened comparing the response in each position. _____

   _____

   B. Which directions in a position are stable? _____

   _____

   C. Explain. _____

   _____

8. Analyze shoulder flexion as if it were a lever system. In the sitting position, move your arm through full shoulder flexion range of motion.

    A. The starting range of motion is _____°, and the ending range of motion is _____°.

    B. What is the "axis" of the motion? _____

    C. Is the movement with or against gravity? _____

    D. Is gravity or muscle the "force" producing the movement? _____

    E. Is gravity or muscle the "resistance" to the movement? _____

    F. Which major muscle group is the agonist? _____

    G. Which major muscle group is the antagonist? _____

    H. Is the agonist acting to overcome gravity or to slow down gravity? _____

    I. Is the agonist performing a concentric or an eccentric contraction? _____

    J. Is the antagonist contracting? _____

    K. Is this an open or closed kinetic chain activity? _____

9. Analyze shoulder extension from full flexion as if it were a lever system. In the sitting position, extend (lower) your arm from full shoulder flexion.

    A. The starting range of motion is _____°, and the ending range of motion is _____°.

    B. What is the "axis" of the motion? _____

    C. Is the movement with or against gravity? _____

    D. Is gravity or the muscle the "force" producing the movement? _____

    E. Is gravity or the muscle the "resistance" to the movement? _____

    F. Which major muscle group is the agonist? _____

    G. Which major muscle group is the antagonist? _____

    H. Is the agonist acting to overcome gravity or to slow down gravity? _____

    I. Is the agonist performing a concentric or an eccentric contraction? _____

    J. Is the antagonist contracting? _____

    K. Is this an open or closed kinetic chain activity? _____

10. Analyze shoulder flexion as if it were a lever system. In the supine position, flex your arm through full shoulder flexion range of motion. ATTENTION: the effect of gravity on the movement of shoulder flexion varies throughout the range.

    First phase: In supine, move the arm from a position next to the body until the hand is pointing to the ceiling.

    A. The starting range of motion is _____°, and the ending range of motion is _____°.

    B. What is the "axis" of the motion? _____

    C. Is the movement with or against gravity? _____

    D. Is gravity or the muscle the "force" producing the movement? _____

    E. Is gravity or the muscle the "resistance" to the movement? _____

    F. Which major muscle group is the agonist? _____

    G. Which major muscle group is the antagonist? _____

    H. Is the agonist acting to overcome gravity or to slow down gravity? _____

I. Is the agonist performing a concentric or an eccentric contraction? _____

J. Is the antagonist contracting? _____

K. Is this an open or closed kinetic chain activity? _____

Second phase: In supine, move the arm from the hand pointing to the ceiling to the end of the range of motion.

A. The starting range of motion is _____°, and the ending range of motion is _____°.

B. What is the "axis" of the motion? _____

C. Is the movement with or against gravity? _____

D. Is gravity or the muscle the "force" producing the movement? _____

E. Is gravity or the muscle the "resistance" to the movement? _____

F. Which major muscle group is the agonist? _____

G. Which major muscle group is the antagonist? _____

H. Is the agonist acting to overcome gravity or to slow down gravity? _____

I. Is the agonist performing a concentric or an eccentric contraction? _____

J. Is the antagonist contracting? _____

K. Is this an open or closed kinetic chain activity? _____

11. Analyze shoulder extension from full flexion as if it were a lever system. In the supine position, extend (lower) your arm from full shoulder flexion. ATTENTION: the effect of gravity on the movement of shoulder extension varies throughout the range.

First phase: In supine, move the arm from full flexion until the hand is pointing to the ceiling.

A. The starting range of motion is _____°, and the ending range of motion is _____°.

B. What is the "axis" of the motion? _____

C. Is the movement with or against gravity? _____

D. Is gravity or the muscle the "force" producing the movement? _____

E. Is gravity or the muscle the "resistance" to the movement? _____

F. Which major muscle group is the agonist? _____

G. Which major muscle group is the antagonist? _____

H. Is the agonist acting to overcome gravity or to slow down gravity? _____

I. Is the agonist performing a concentric or an eccentric contraction? _____

J. Is the antagonist contracting? _____

K. Is this an open or closed kinetic chain activity? _____

Second phase: In supine, move the arm from the hand pointing to the ceiling to a position next to the body.

A. The starting range of motion is _____°, and the ending range of motion is _____°.

B. What is the "axis" of the motion? _____

C. Is the movement with or against gravity? _____

D. Is gravity or the muscle the "force" producing the movement? _____

E. Is gravity or the muscle the "resistance" to the movement? _____

F. Which major muscle group is the agonist? _____

G. Which major muscle group is the antagonist? _____

H. Is the agonist acting to overcome gravity or to slow down gravity? _____

I. Is the agonist performing a concentric or an eccentric contraction? _____

J. Is the antagonist contracting? _____

K. Is this an open or closed kinetic chain activity? _____

■ ■ ■ Post-Lab Questions

Student's Name_____ Date Due _____

After you have completed the Worksheets and Lab Activities, answer the following questions without using your book or notes. When finished, check your answers.

1. What can be stated about BOS and COG that describe a stable object?

_____

_____

2. For each class of lever, identify the relationship of the axis, resistance arm, and force arm and name a tool that uses that lever class.

   A. 1st class ____ ____ ____ _____

   B. 2nd class ____ ____ ____ _____

   C. 3rd class ____ ____ ____ _____

3. Describe how the angle of pull of the elbow flexors creates angular forces, stabilizing forces, and dislocating forces.

_____

_____

4. Moment arm or torque arm is the _____ distance from the line of action of the

   _____ to the _____ of rotation. The moment arm of a muscle is greatest

   when the line of pull of a muscle is at _____°.

5. Standing, perform hip flexion first with the knee flexed and second with knee extended.

   Which takes more hip flexor strength? _____ With knee flexed. _____
   With knee extended.

   Why?

_____

_____

6. A person riding a bus is standing facing the front of the bus. How should the person place his or her feet to maintain balance when the bus:

   A. Stops?

   _____

   B. Turns a corner?

   _____

7. What happens to the COG when a person holds a 20-pound weight in the left hand?

   _____

   To compensate for the 20-pound weight, in which direction does a person shift the COG?

   _____

8. When the force arm is longer than the resistance arm, is it easier or harder to move?

   _____

Clinical Kinesiology and Anatomy of the Upper Extremities

Shoulder Girdle

■ ■ ■ Worksheets

Student's Name _____ Date Due _____

Complete the following questions prior to lab class.

1. In the table, indicate which bones make up each of the structures.

Structures	Scapula	Clavicle	Sternum	Rib Cage	Humerus
Shoulder complex					
Scapulothoracic articulation					
Shoulder girdle					
Shoulder joint					

2. Define the following terms:

   Scapulohumeral rhythm:

   _____

   _____

   Reversal of muscle action:

   _____

   _____

3. Label Figures 8-1 through 8-3 with the following terms:

SCAPULA: Superior angle   Inferior angle
            Vertebral border   Axillary border
            Spine   Coracoid process
            Acromion process   Glenoid fossa

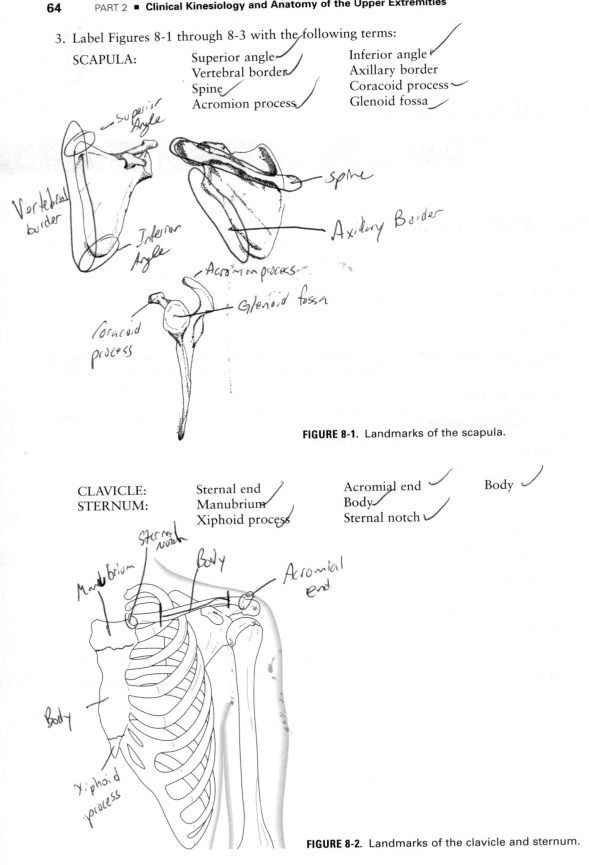

FIGURE 8-1. Landmarks of the scapula.

CLAVICLE: Sternal end   Acromial end   Body
STERNUM: Manubrium   Body
            Xiphoid process   Sternal notch

FIGURE 8-2. Landmarks of the clavicle and sternum.

SKULL: Occipital protuberance
VERTEBRA: Spinous process   Transverse process

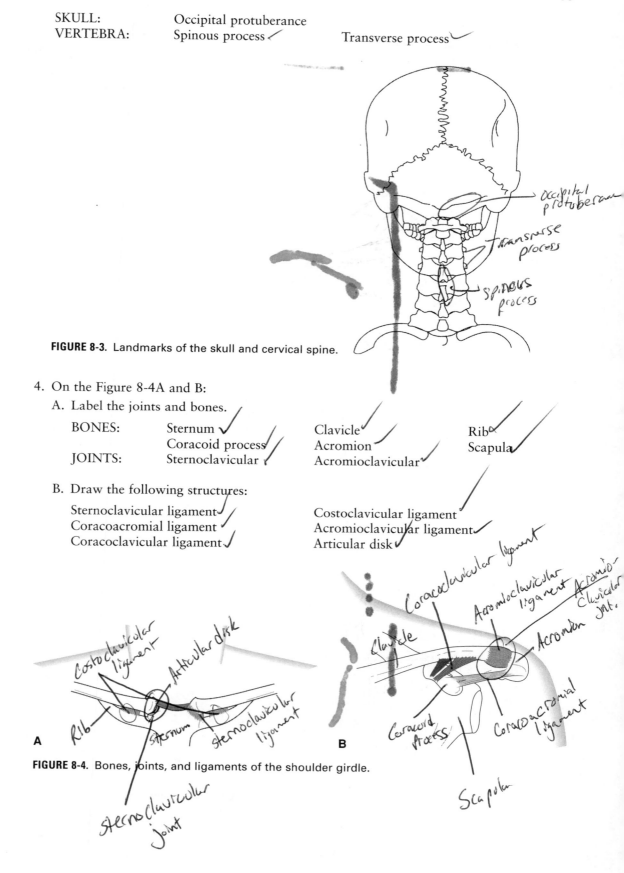

FIGURE 8-3. Landmarks of the skull and cervical spine.

4. On the Figure 8-4A and B:
   A. Label the joints and bones.

   BONES: Sternum   Clavicle   Rib
               Coracoid process   Acromion   Scapula
   JOINTS: Sternoclavicular   Acromioclavicular

   B. Draw the following structures:

   Sternoclavicular ligament   Costoclavicular ligament
   Coracoacromial ligament   Acromioclavicular ligament
   Coracoclavicular ligament   Articular disk

FIGURE 8-4. Bones, joints, and ligaments of the shoulder girdle.

5. On Figures 8-5 through 8-8:

A. Label the origin and insertion of the following muscles:
   Color the origin in red and the insertion in blue.

B. Join the origin and insertion to show the line of pull.

Upper Trapezius Muscle

O – Occipital Bone, nuchal ligament on cervical spinous process

I – Outer third of clavicle, acromion process

A – Scapular elevation & upward rot.

N – Spinal accessory (cranial Nerve XI)
   C3/C4 sensory component.

see pg. 100

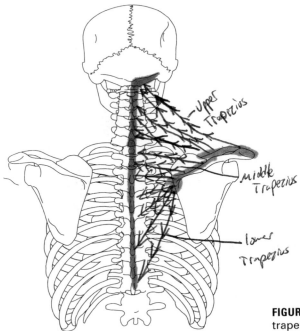

FIGURE 8-5. Upper, middle, and lower trapezius.

see pg. 101

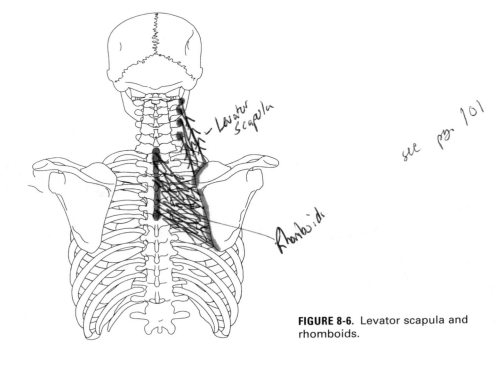

FIGURE 8-6. Levator scapula and rhomboids.

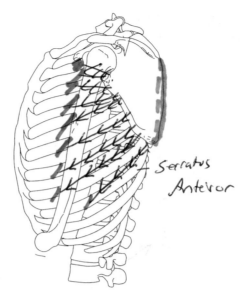

see pg. 107

FIGURE 8-7. Serratus anterior.

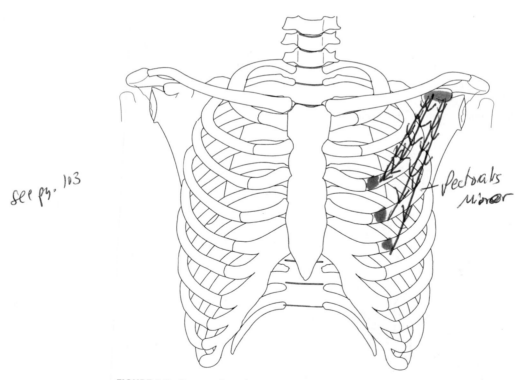

see pg. 103

FIGURE 8-8. Pectoralis minor.

6. Draw in the muscles that make up the force couples acting on the scapula to produce upward rotation in Figure 8-9 and downward rotation in Figure 8-10. Label the muscles involved.

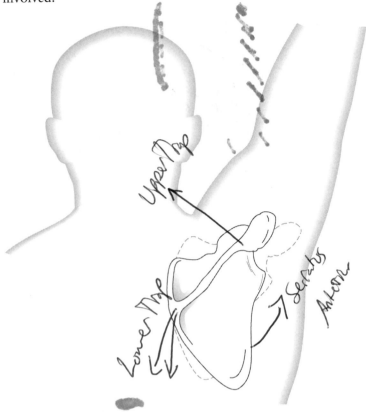

FIGURE 8-9. Upward rotation of the scapula.

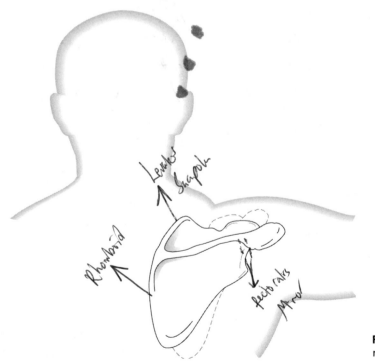

FIGURE 8-10. Downward rotation of the scapula.

7. Identify the shoulder girdle motion illustrated in Figure 8-11.

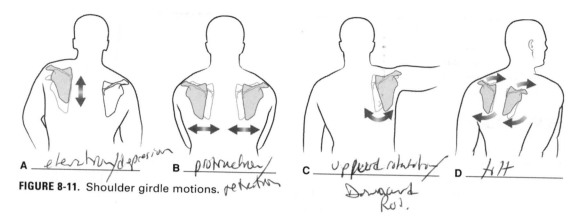

A ___elevation/depression___   B ___protraction___   C ___upward rotation___ D ___tilt___

FIGURE 8-11. Shoulder girdle motions. _retraction_   _Downward Rot._

8. Match each ligament or structure to the appropriate function. There may be more than one correct answer, and answers may be used more than once.

_____ Connects sternum to clavicle	A. Sternoclavicular ligament
_____ Connects first rib to clavicle	B. Costoclavicular ligament
_____ Connects clavicles	C. Articular disk
_____ Connects scapula to clavicle	D. Interclavicular ligament
_____ Reinforces the capsule	E. Acromioclavicular ligament
_____ Limits clavicular elevation	F. Coracoacromial ligament
_____ Acts as a shock absorber	
_____ Limits clavicular depression	
_____ Serves as roof over humeral head	
_____ Provides protective arch	

9. For each motion listed, check the muscles that are the major contributors to the motion.

Motions	Upper Trapezius	Middle Trapezius	Lower Trapezius	Rhomboids	Serratus Anterior	Pectoralis Minor	Levator Scapula
Elevation							
Depression							
Protraction							
Retraction							
Upward rotation							
Downward rotation							

10. At the sternoclavicular joint, identify which surface is concave and which is convex.

Joint	Concave	Convex
Sternoclavicular		

■ ■ ■ Lab Activities

Student's Name _____ Date Due _____

1. Perform the motions of the shoulder girdle with your partner.

   A. Perform a motion and your partner names the motion you performed.

   B. Your partner calls a motion and you perform that motion.

2. On the skeleton, anatomical models, and at least one partner, locate, palpate, and observe the following structures. The reference position is the anatomical position. Having pictures for reference is helpful when trying to find structures. Not all structures are palpable on your partner.

Sternum:	Located midline of the anterior chest wall. 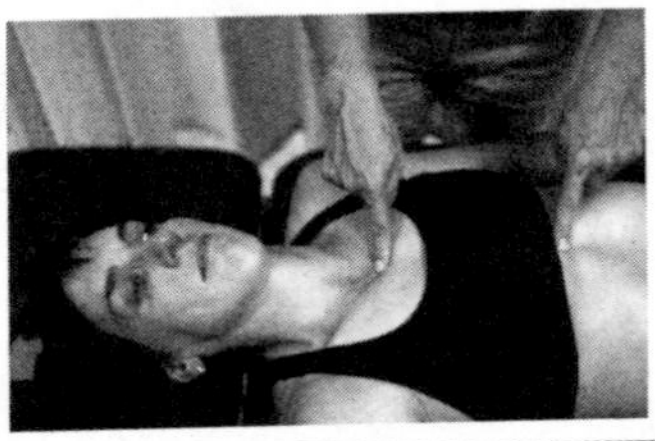 **FIGURE 8-12**. Palpation of the sternum.
Manubrium:	The superior portion of the sternum. 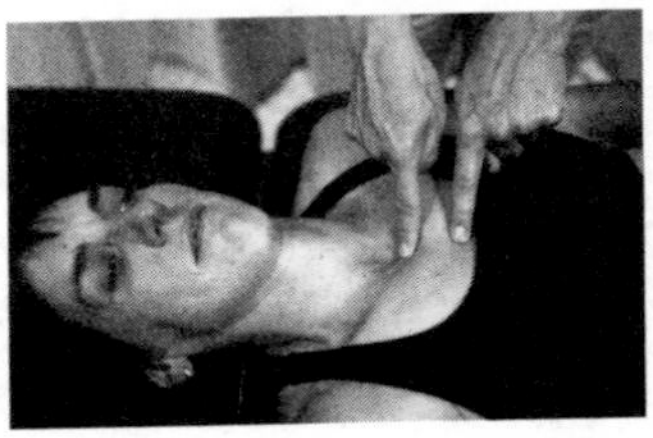 **FIGURE 8-13**. Palpation of the manubrium.
Body:	The middle and largest portion of the sternum. 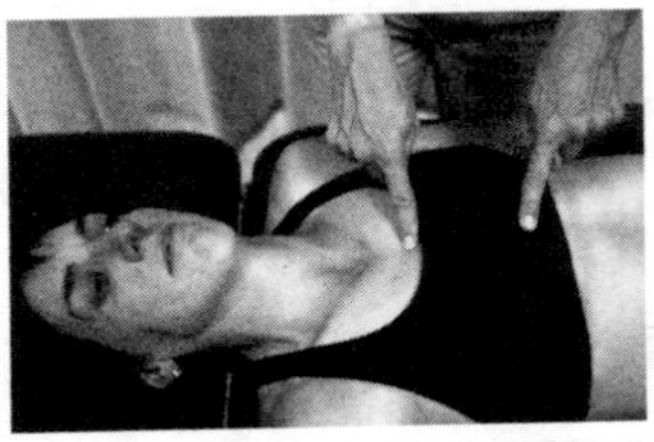 **FIGURE 8-14**. Palpation of the body of the sternum.

(Continued...)

Xiphoid process:	The inferior portion of the sternum. The most inferior part of the xiphoid process is called the tip of the xiphoid.

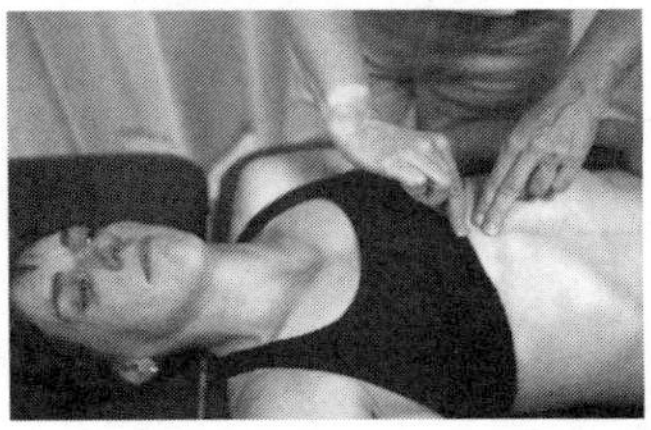

FIGURE 8-15. Palpation of the xiphoid process.

Sternal notch:	The indentation at the top of the manubrium formed by the right and left clavicles and the manubrium. Palpate the sternum starting at the sternal notch, and moving inferiorly palpating in turn the manubrium, body, and xiphoid process.

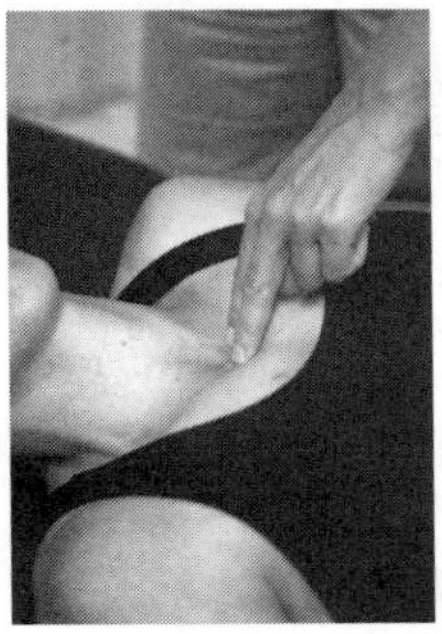

FIGURE 8-16. Palpation of the sternal notch.

Clavicle:	Located on the anterior surface of the trunk, superior and lateral to the sternum. Palpate starting at the sternal notch and moving horizontally, laterally, and posteriorly along the clavicle to the acromioclavicular joint. Note that the medial two-thirds is convex and the lateral one-third is concave.

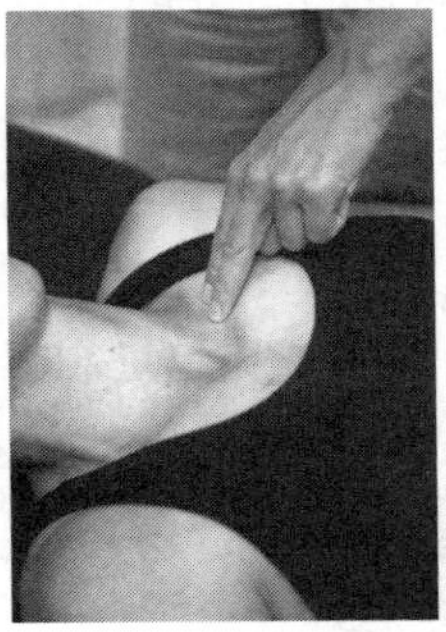

FIGURE 8-17. Palpation of the clavicle.

Scapula:	Located superiorly on the posterior surface of the trunk between T2 and T7.
Vertebral border:	The medial edge of the scapula, which is approximately parallel to the vertebral column. Palpate from superior to inferior. Medially rotating the shoulder joint by placing the hand on the low back often causes the vertebral border to move away from the thorax.

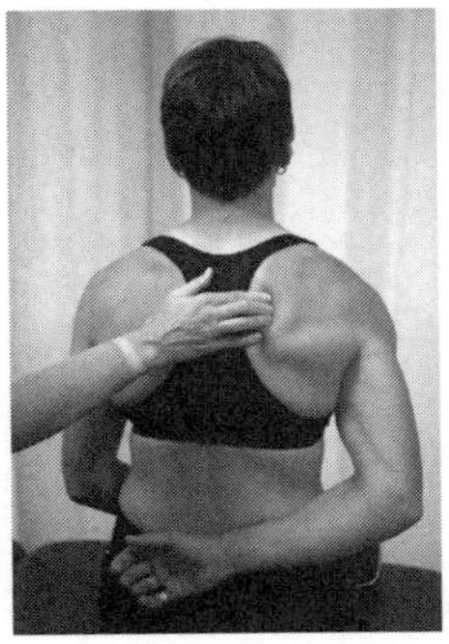

FIGURE 8-18. Palpation of the vertebral border.

(Continued...)

Inferior angle:	The inferior point of the scapula where the vertebral and axillary borders meet.

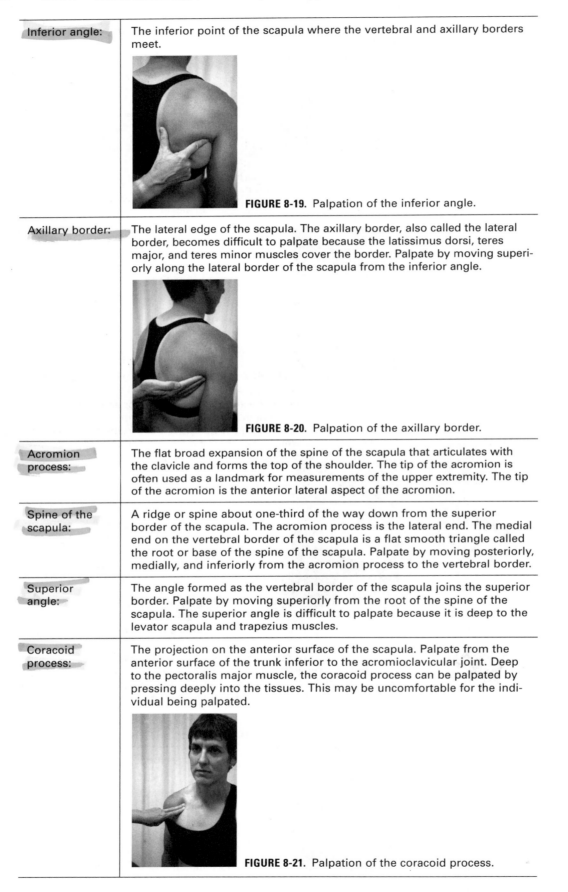

FIGURE 8-19. Palpation of the inferior angle.

Axillary border:	The lateral edge of the scapula. The axillary border, also called the lateral border, becomes difficult to palpate because the latissimus dorsi, teres major, and teres minor muscles cover the border. Palpate by moving superiorly along the lateral border of the scapula from the inferior angle.

FIGURE 8-20. Palpation of the axillary border.

Acromion process:	The flat broad expansion of the spine of the scapula that articulates with the clavicle and forms the top of the shoulder. The tip of the acromion is often used as a landmark for measurements of the upper extremity. The tip of the acromion is the anterior lateral aspect of the acromion.
Spine of the scapula:	A ridge or spine about one-third of the way down from the superior border of the scapula. The acromion process is the lateral end. The medial end on the vertebral border of the scapula is a flat smooth triangle called the root or base of the spine of the scapula. Palpate by moving posteriorly, medially, and inferiorly from the acromion process to the vertebral border.
Superior angle:	The angle formed as the vertebral border of the scapula joins the superior border. Palpate by moving superiorly from the root of the spine of the scapula. The superior angle is difficult to palpate because it is deep to the levator scapula and trapezius muscles.
Coracoid process:	The projection on the anterior surface of the scapula. Palpate from the anterior surface of the trunk inferior to the acromioclavicular joint. Deep to the pectoralis major muscle, the coracoid process can be palpated by pressing deeply into the tissues. This may be uncomfortable for the individual being palpated.

FIGURE 8-21. Palpation of the coracoid process.

3. Locate the following muscles on the skeleton, anatomical models, and on at least one partner.

   A. Locate the origin and insertion of the muscle on the skeleton.

   B. Stretch a large rubber band taut by placing one end at the origin and the other end at the insertion of the muscle.

   C. Perform the motion that the muscle does and observe how the rubber band becomes less taut, similar to the muscle shortening as it contracts.

   D. Perform the opposite motion and observe how the rubber band becomes more taut and elongated, simulating the muscle being stretched.

   E. After locating the muscle on the skeleton, locate the muscle on your partner. The position described for locating the muscle on your partner is the manual muscle test position for a fair or better grade of muscle strength. Not all origins, insertions, and muscle bellies can be palpated on your partner.

   F. When possible, palpate the origin, insertion, and muscle belly of each muscle by:

   1) Placing your fingers on the origin and insertion and asking your partner to contract the muscle.

   2) Moving your fingers from the origin to the insertion over the contracting muscle.

   3) Asking your partner to relax the muscle, and again moving your fingers from the origin to the insertion over the muscle.

   G. In the following tables, the information needed to palpate each muscle is provided. The information includes position of the person, origin and insertion of the muscle, the line of pull of the muscle, the muscle's action, instructions to give to the person to make the muscle contract, and, finally, information on the best location to palpate the muscle.

Sitting Position

UPPER TRAPEZIUS:	Located superficially on the posterior thorax.
	FIGURE 8-22. Palpation of the upper trapezius.
Position of person:	Sit facing away from the examiner with hands relaxed in the lap.
Origin:	Occipital protuberance and nuchal ligament of cervical spinous processes.
Insertion:	Outer third of clavicle and acromion process.
Line of pull:	Diagonal (more vertical than horizontal).
Muscle action:	Prime mover in scapular elevation and upward rotation, and only assistive in scapular retraction.
Palpate:	On the superior and posterior aspect of the thorax above the scapula.
Instructions to person:	Shrug or raise your shoulder toward your ear.

(Continued...)

Sitting Position (continued)

LEVATOR SCAPULA:	Located on the posterior thorax deep to the upper trapezius. Its location and the fact that is has similar action to the upper trapezius makes it difficult to palpate.
Position of person:	Sit facing away from the examiner with the hands relaxed in the lap.
Origin:	Transverse processes of C1–C4 vertebrae.
Insertion:	Vertebral border of scapula between the superior angle and the root of the spine.
Line of pull:	Diagonal line of pull that is mostly vertical.
Muscle action:	Prime mover for scapular elevation and downward rotation, and assistive in scapular retraction.
Palpate:	On the posterior surface of the thorax at the superior angle of the scapula.
Instructions to person:	Shrug your shoulder toward your ear.
PECTORALIS MINOR:	Located on the anterior chest wall deep to the pectoralis major.

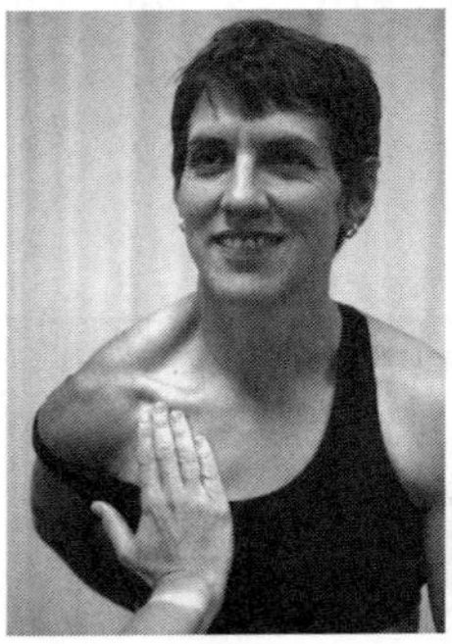

FIGURE 8-23. Palpation of the pectoralis minor.

Position of person:	Sit facing the examiner with the hand of the side being palpated resting on the low back.
Origin:	Anterior medial outer surfaces of ribs 3–5.
Insertion:	Coracoid process of the scapula.
Line of pull:	Diagonal (downward pull is vertical).
Muscle action:	Prime mover for scapular depression, downward rotation, and tilt.
Palpate:	Below the coracoid process.
Instructions to person:	Lift your hand off your low back.

(Continued...)

SERRATUS ANTERIOR:	Located on the anterior lateral chest wall deep to the latissimus dorsi laterally and deep to the scapula posteriorly. 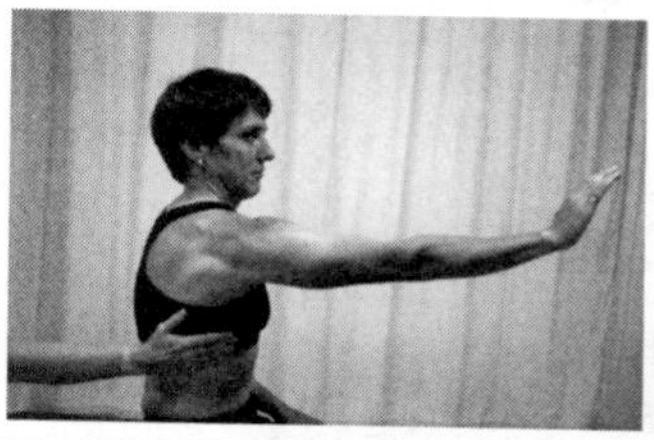 **FIGURE 8-24.** Palpation of the serratus anterior.
Position of person:	Sit with the shoulder flexed to 90°.
Origin:	Lateral aspects of first eight ribs.
Insertion:	Anterior surface of the vertebral border of the scapula.
Line of pull:	Horizontal.
Muscle action:	Prime mover for scapular protraction and upward rotation.
Palpate:	On the anterior lateral aspect of the chest wall.
Instructions to person:	Reach forward with your shoulder flexed by moving your scapula.

Prone Position

LOWER TRAPEZIUS:	Located superficially on the posterior thorax.
Position of person:	Lie prone with the shoulder abducted to approximately 145° (in line with the fibers of the muscle). 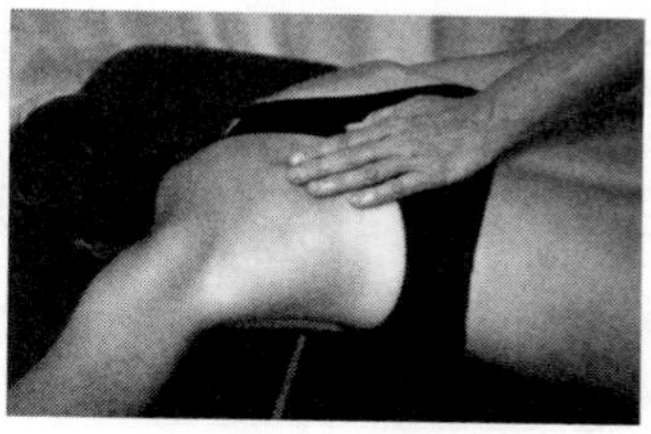 **FIGURE 8-25.** Palpation of the lower trapezius.
Origin:	Spinous processes of middle and lower thoracic vertebrae.
Insertion:	Base of the spine of the scapula.
Line of pull:	Diagonal (downward).
Muscle action:	Prime mover for scapular depression and upward rotation and assistive in retraction.
Palpate:	The muscle belly inferior and medial to the insertion.
Instructions to person:	Lift your arm off the table toward the ceiling.

(*Continued...*)

Prone Position (continued)

MIDDLE TRAPEZIUS:	Located superficially on the posterior thorax. **FIGURE 8-26.** Palpation of the middle trapezius.
Position of person:	Lie prone with shoulder abducted to 90° and the elbow flexed to 90°. The forearm should be hanging over the edge of the table.
Origin:	Spinous processes of C7–T3.
Insertion:	Medial aspect of the acromion process and spine of the scapula.
Line of pull:	Horizontal.
Muscle action:	Prime mover for scapular retraction and assistive for upward rotation.
Palpate:	Lateral to the origin.
Instructions to person:	Lift your upper arm off the table toward the ceiling.
RHOMBOIDS:	Located on the posterior thorax deep to the trapezius.
Position of person:	Lie prone with hand resting on the low back.
Origin:	Spinous processes of C7–T5 vertebrae.
Insertion:	Vertebral border of scapula between the spine and the inferior angle of the spine.
Line of pull:	Diagonal.
Muscle action:	Prime mover in scapular retraction, elevation, and downward rotation.
Palpate:	Medial to the vertebral border of the scapula.
Instructions to person:	Lift your hand off your low back toward the ceiling.

4. Scapular motion
   A. Observe scapular motion as your partner flexes his or her shoulder. List the scapular motion(s) you observed.

   _____

   _____

B. Place one hand along the vertebral border. Palpate the movement of the scapula as your partner repeats shoulder flexion. Describe what you felt.

_____

_____

C. Stabilize the scapula to prevent its movement as your partner attempts shoulder flexion. Describe what you observed.

_____

_____

5. Observe and palpate as your partner performs shoulder abduction starting in the anatomical position.

A. Describe the movements of the scapula and humerus in relation to one another.

_____

_____

B. What is the name given to this combination of movements?

_____

_____

6. Work in groups of at least three members. Have one person stand erect. Have the second partner place a heavy weight in the first person's right hand, while the third member of the group palpates right shoulder girdle musculature.

A. What happened to the shoulder girdle (e.g., elevation or depression) on the side holding the weight?

_____

B. Name any shoulder girdle musculature that contracted in response to the weight.

_____

C. Is the weight exerting _____ traction or _____ approximation on the shoulder girdle? (Select one)

D. Is this _____ an open or _____ a closed kinetic chain activity? (Select one)

E. Perform shoulder elevation of the side holding the weight.

Are the shoulder elevator muscles _____ overcoming gravity or _____ slowing down gravity? (Select one)

Are the muscles performing _____ concentric or _____ eccentric contractions? (Select one)

7. A. When your partner assumes the hands-and-knees position, with the shoulders and back relaxed, what position do your partner's scapulas assume?

_____ Neutral   _____ Protracted   _____ Retracted   _____ Winged

B. Is this _____ an open or _____ a closed kinetic chain activity? (Select one)

■ ■ ■ Post-Lab Questions

Student's Name _____ Date Due _____

After you have completed the Worksheets and Lab Activities, answer the following questions without using your book or notes. When finished, check your answers.

1. List the muscle(s) of the shoulder girdle that attach to the ribs.

   _____

2. List the muscle(s) of the shoulder girdle that attach to the vertebral border of the scapula.

   _____

3. List the muscle(s) of the shoulder girdle that attach to the skull.

   _____

4. List the muscle(s) of the shoulder girdle that attach to the vertebral column.

   _____

5. List the muscle(s) of the shoulder girdle that attach to the clavicle.

   _____

6. List the joints that make up the shoulder girdle.

   _____

   _____

7. Why is the scapulothoracic joint not a true joint?

   _____

   _____

8. What is the result of limited sternoclavicular motion on shoulder girdle motion?

   _____

   _____

9. Using the following descriptive terminology, fill in the blanks in the following sentences. Use each term once.

Medial	Anterior	Superior	Deep
Lateral	Posterior	Inferior	Superficial

   A. The spine is on the _____ surface of the scapula.

   B. The vertebral border is on the _____ side of the scapula.

   C. The glenoid fossa is on the _____ aspect of the scapula.

   D. The xiphoid process is _____ to the body of the sternum.

   E. The rhomboid muscles are located _____ to the trapezius.

   F. The coracoid process is on the _____ surface of the scapula.

   G. The upper trapezius muscle is _____ to the levator scapula.

   H. The clavicle is _____ to the first rib.

10. Identify the following muscles:

    A. Attaches to the coracoid process: _____

    B. Attaches to the vertebral border of the scapula:

        1) On the posterior surface: _____

        2) On the anterior surface: _____

    C. Attaches to the superior angle of the scapula: _____

    D. Attaches to the spine of the scapula: _____

    E. Attaches at the base of the scapular spine: _____

    F. Attaches on the transverse processes of the vertebra: _____

    G. Attaches on the spinous process of the vertebra: _____

11. Identify the following muscles according to their locations on the body:

    A. Which muscle is located between the rib cage and the scapula?

    _____

    B. Which muscle lies deep to the pectoralis major?

    _____

    C. Which muscle is the most superficial on the posterior upper back?

    _____

12. Name the shoulder girdle muscle innervated by a cranial nerve:

    _____

    Name the cranial nerve:

    _____

Shoulder Joint

■ ■ ■ Worksheets

Student's Name _____ Date Due _____

Complete the following questions prior to lab class.

1. On Figures 9-1A and B, label the following landmarks:

   SCAPULA: Glenoid fossa   Labrum
               Subscapular fossa   Infraspinous fossa
               Supraspinous fossa   Axillary border
               Acromion process   Vertebral border
   HUMERUS: Head   Surgical neck
               Anatomical neck   Shaft
               Greater tubercle   Lesser tubercle
               Deltoid tuberosity   Bicipital groove

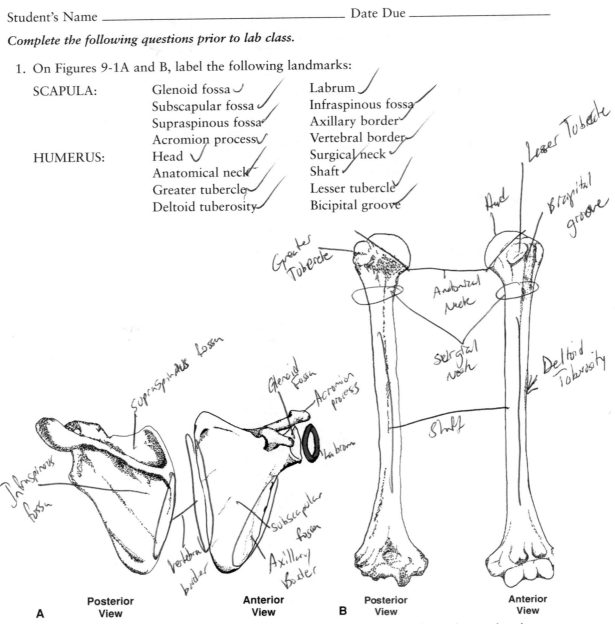

| A | Posterior View | Anterior View | B | Posterior View | Anterior View |

FIGURE 9-1 *(A)* Scapula, anterior and posterior view. *(B)* Humerus, anterior and posterior view.

2. On Figure 9-2:

    A. Label the shoulder joint and bones.

    B. Label the following structures:

        Glenohumeral ligaments   Coracohumeral ligament

        Greater tubercle   Capsule

        Tendon of long head of biceps

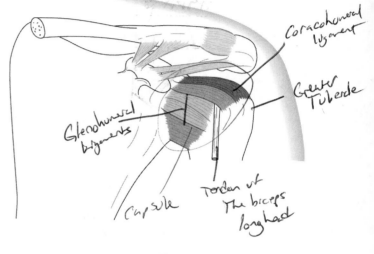

FIGURE 9-2. Shoulder ligaments.

3. On Figures 9-3 through 9-7:

    A. Label the origin and insertion of the muscles listed.

    B. Join the origin and insertion to show the line of pull.

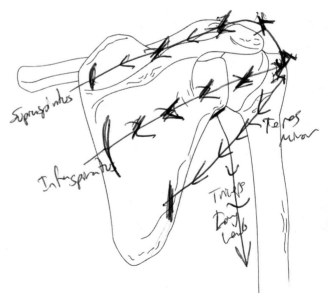

FIGURE 9-3. Supraspinatus, infraspinatus, teres minor, and triceps-long head proximal attachment.

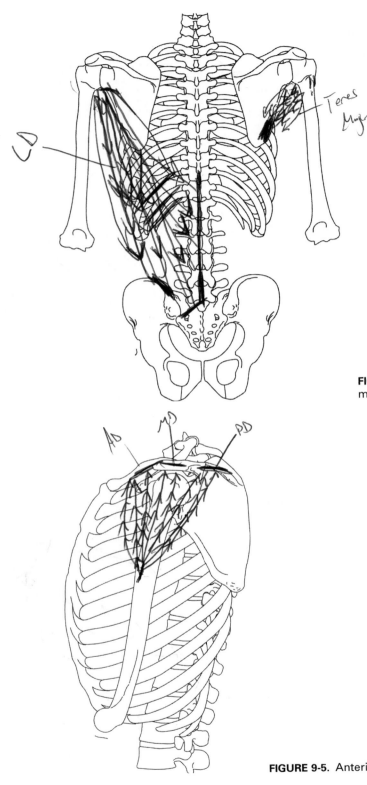

FIGURE 9-4. Latissimus dorsi, teres major.

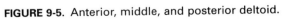

FIGURE 9-5. Anterior, middle, and posterior deltoid.

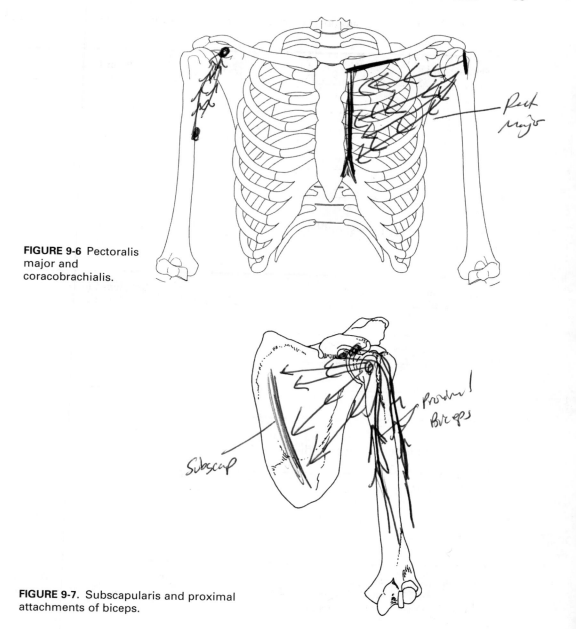

FIGURE 9-6 Pectoralis major and coracobrachialis.

FIGURE 9-7. Subscapularis and proximal attachments of biceps.

4. Describe the role of scapulohumeral rhythm and the "inchworm effect" to maintaining the effectiveness of the shoulder muscles.

_____

_____

5. Distinguish between the shoulder joint and the shoulder girdle by *listing the bones* of each.

Shoulder Joint	Shoulder Girdle

6. Distinguish between the shoulder joint and the shoulder girdle by *listing the motions* available at each.

Shoulder Joint	Shoulder Girdle

7. For the shoulder joint, identify the:
   A. Type of joint: _____
   B. Shape of the joint: _____

8. For the motions available at the shoulder joint, indicate in which plane and about which axis motion occurs.

Motions	Plane	Axis
Flexion/Extension/Hyperextension		
Abduction/Adduction		
Medial/Lateral Rotation		

9. Identify which surface of the shoulder joint is concave and which is convex.

Joint	Concave	Convex
Shoulder joint		

10. For the shoulder joint, provide the close-packed position and the loose-packed position. (Refer to Chapter 4.)

Joint	Close-Packed	Loose-Packed
Shoulder		

11. Match each ligament and structure to the appropriate function or characteristic. Use each answer once.

_____ Provides attachment for the latissimus dorsi muscle

_____ Deepens the joint

_____ Keeps the humeral head rotating in contact with the glenoid fossa

_____ Surrounds the joint

_____ Strengthens the upper part of the joint capsule

_____ Decreases friction between the deltoid muscle and the joint capsule

_____ Decreases friction between the acromion process, the coracoacromial ligament, and the joint capsule

A. Coracohumeral ligament

B. Glenoid labrum

C. Subdeltoid bursa

D. Subacromial bursa

E. Rotator cuff

F. Thoracolumbar fascia

G. Joint capsule

12. For each motion listed, check the muscle(s) that are major contributors to the motion.

Motion	Anterior Deltoid	Middle Deltoid	Posterior Deltoid	Supraspinatus	Coracobrachialis	Subscapularis
Flexion						
Extension						
Hyperextension						
Medial rotation						
Lateral rotation						
Abduction						
Adduction						
Horizontal abduction						
Horizontal adduction						

Motion	Pectoralis Major Clavicular	Pectoralis Major Sternal	Latissimus Dorsi	Teres Major	Teres Minor	Infraspinatus
Flexion						
Extension						
Hyperextension						
Medial rotation						
Lateral rotation						
Abduction						
Adduction						
Horizontal abduction						
Horizontal adduction						

13. Describe the function of the rotator cuff muscles during shoulder flexion or abduction.

_____

_____

14. A. Which major nerve unit is located in the axilla?

_____

  B. That nerve unit is where in relation to the head of the humerus:

  _____ Anterior _____ Posterior _____ Superior _____ Inferior

  C. What major blood vessel is close to this nerve unit? _____

15. Diagram the lever that describes *abduction of the shoulder joint* performed in standing and starting in the anatomical position.
  A. Draw a stick figure performing shoulder abduction from the anatomical position.
  B. Draw arrows to indicate the direction of the movement, the direction of the pull of the muscle, and the direction of gravity.
  C. Label the arrow that represents force with "F" and the arrow that represents resistance with "R".

16. Analyze the activity of shoulder abduction diagrammed in question 15 by answering the following questions:

    A. The starting range of motion is _____ °, and the ending range of motion is _____ °.

    B. What is the "axis" of the motion? _____

    C. Is the movement with or against gravity? _____

    D. Is gravity or muscle the "force" producing the movement? _____

    E. Is gravity or muscle the "resistance" to the movement? _____

    F. Which major muscle group is the agonist? _____

    G. Which major muscle group is the antagonist? _____

    H. Is the agonist acting to overcome gravity or to slow down gravity? _____

    I. Is the agonist performing a concentric or an eccentric contraction? _____

    J. Is the antagonist contracting? _____

    K. Is this an open or closed kinetic chain activity? _____

■ ■ ■ Lab Activities

Student's Name _____ Date Due _____

1. Perform the motions of the shoulder joint with your partner.
    A. Perform a motion and your partner names the motion you performed.
    B. Your partner states a motion and you perform that motion.

2. Using worksheets question 8 for reference, for each of the motions available at the shoulder joint:
    A. Place your open left hand in the correct orientation to represent the plane of a motion.
    B. Place your right index finger to indicate the axis of that plane of motion.

3. Knowing the amount of motion at a joint is important for planning interventions and determining change. The normal amount of motion for each plane of motion at a joint is known. Being able to estimate the amount of joint motion present is useful. The anatomical position is considered the 0° position for most joints and is the starting position for measuring the amount of motion available in each plane. To begin to estimate the amount of joint motion, identify the landmark degrees of 0°, 45°, 90°, 135°, and 180°. A right angle is 90°. Halfway between 0° and 90° is 45°; 135° is halfway between 90° and 180°.

    A. Move the arms of the goniometer to each of the following angles 0°, 45°, 90°, 135°, and 180°.

    B. Without using a goniometer, place your partner's arm in 0°, 45°, 90°, 135°, and 180° of shoulder flexion.

C. For each of the motions available at the shoulder joint, estimate the degrees of motion available by checking the box that *most closely* describes that motion. (Do not use a goniometer.)

Motions	0°–45°	46°–90°	91°–135°	136°–180°
Flexion				
Hyperextension				
Abduction				
Horizontal abduction*				
Horizontal adduction*				
Medial rotation**				
Lateral rotation**				

*Starting position: shoulder abducted to 90°.
**Starting position: elbow flexed to 90°.

4. Being able to determine the end feel of a joint is part of an examination of a joint. With your partner in sitting or supine, move the shoulder joint through the available ROM. At the end of the ROM in each plane of motion observe the end feel. Repeat with several people. (Refer to Chapter 4 for descriptions of end feel.)

   What end feel(s) for motions of the shoulder joint did you observe?

   _____ Bony   _____ Capsular   _____ Soft   _____ Empty

5. On the skeleton, anatomical models, and at least one partner, locate, palpate, and observe the following structures. The reference position is the anatomical position. Having pictures for reference is helpful when trying to find structures. Not all structures are palpable on your partner.

   SCAPULA: Some of the landmarks on the scapula were described in the lab on the shoulder girdle, Chapter 8.

Glenoid fossa	A shallow socket on the superior end, lateral side; it articulates with the humerus. Cannot be palpated.
Glenoid labrum	Fibrocartilaginous ring attached to the rim of the glenoid fossa, which deepens the articular cavity. Cannot be palpated.
Subscapular fossa	Includes most of the area on the anterior surface; provides attachment for the subscapularis muscle. Cannot be palpated.
Infraspinous fossa	Area on the posterior surface, below the spine; provides attachment for the infraspinatus muscle. Cannot be palpated.
Supraspinous fossa	Area on the posterior surface, above the spine, providing attachment for the supraspinatus muscle. Cannot be palpated.
Axillary border	Lateral aspect, provides attachment for teres major and teres minor muscles. See Figure 8-20.
Acromion process	Broad, flat area on the superior lateral aspect of the scapula; it provides attachment for the middle deltoid muscle. 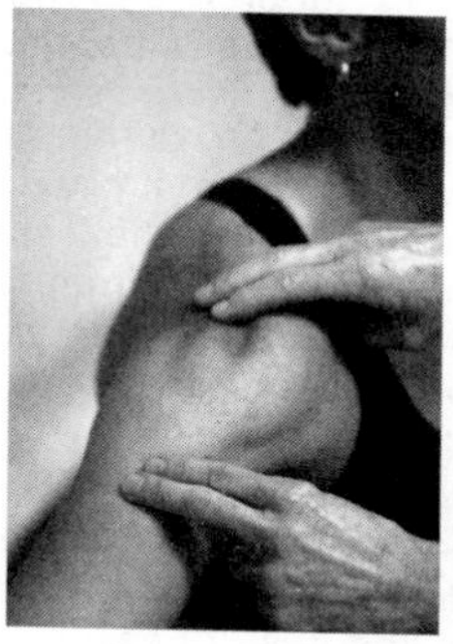 **FIGURE 9-8.** The examiner's right hand is on the acromion process and left hand is on the deltoid tuberosity.

Humerus

Head	Smooth semi-round portion of the proximal end medial aspect of the humerus. The head of the humerus fits in the glenoid fossa to the complete the shoulder joint. The head is palpable when the shoulder joint is laterally rotated. 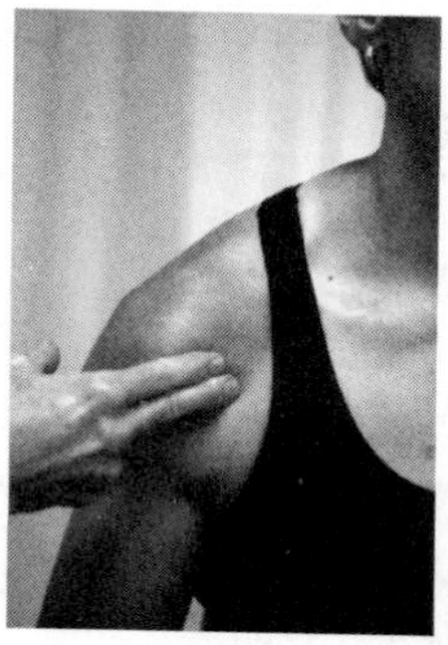 **FIGURE 9-9.** Palpating the head of humerus.
Surgical neck	Slightly constricted area just distal to the tubercles where the head meets the body of the humerus. Cannot be palpated.
Anatomical neck	Circumferential groove separating the head from the tubercles. Cannot be palpated.
Shaft	Extends from the surgical neck proximally to the epicondyles distally. Also known as the body of the humerus.

(Continued...)

Humerus *(continued)*

Greater tubercle	Large projection on the proximal end of the humerus lateral to head and lesser tubercle. It provides attachment for the supraspinatus, infraspinatus, and teres minor muscles. Palpate the greater tubercle on your partner by finding the tip of the acromion process and sliding distally onto the greater tubercle of the humerus. A second method is palpating the proximal anterior surface of the humerus while medially rotating the humerus. This movement causes the greater tubercle to move under your fingers. 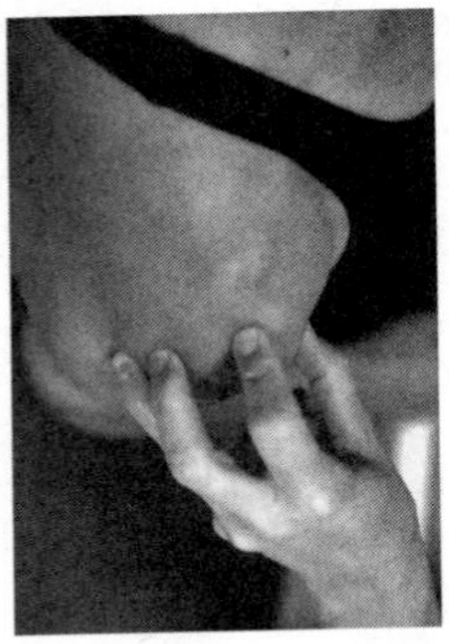 **FIGURE 9-10.** The thumb is on the lesser tubercle and the index finger is on the greater tubercle.
Lesser tubercle	Smaller projection on the proximal anterior surface of the humerus medial to the greater tubercle; it provides attachment for the subscapularis muscle. Palpate the lesser tubercle on your partner by placing your fingers on the proximal anterior surface of the humerus medial to the greater tubercle while laterally rotating the humerus with your other hand. This movement causes the lesser tubercle to move under your fingers.
Deltoid tuberosity	Located laterally at the midpoint of the shaft of the humerus. The deltoid muscle inserts on the deltoid tuberosity. It is not a well-defined structure, and it is not easily palpated. See Figure 9-8.
Bicipital groove	Located between the tubercles on the proximal anterior surface of the humerus. Also called the intertubercular groove. Palpate the bicipital groove on your partner by placing your fingers on the proximal anterior surface of the humerus. Medial and lateral rotation causes the greater and lesser tubercles to move under your fingers. The space between the tubercles is the bicipital groove. The biceps tendon lies in the bicipital groove. Palpation of the groove may produce discomfort when too much pressure is applied. 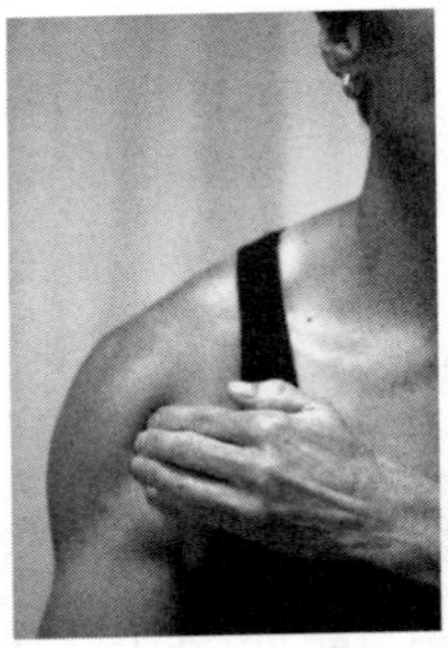 **FIGURE 9-11.** Palpating the bicipital groove.
Bicipital ridges	Also called the lateral and medial lips of the bicipital groove, or the crests of the greater and lesser tubercles. The lateral lip (crest of the greater tubercle) provides attachment for the pectoralis major, and the medial lip (crest of the lesser tubercle) provides attachment for the latissimus dorsi and teres major.

6. Locate the following on the skeleton, anatomical models, and at least one partner:

   A. Locate the origin and insertion of the muscle on the skeleton.

   B. Stretch a large rubber band taut by placing one end at the origin and the other end at the insertion of the muscle on the skeleton.

   C. Perform the motion that the muscle does and observe how the rubber band becomes less taut and shorter, similar to the muscle shortening as it contracts.

   D. Perform the opposite motion and observe how the rubber band becomes more taut and longer, similar to the muscle lengthening as it is being stretched.

   E. After locating the muscle on the skeleton, locate the muscle on your partner. The position described for locating the muscle on your partner is the manual muscle test position for a fair or better grade of muscle strength. Not all origins, insertions, and muscle bellies can be palpated on your partner.

   F. When possible, palpate the origin, insertion, and muscle belly of each muscle by:

      1) Placing your fingers on the origin and insertion and asking your partner to contract the muscle.

      2) Moving your fingers from the origin to the insertion over the contracting muscle.

      3) Asking your partner to relax the muscle and again moving your fingers from the origin to the insertion over the muscle.

   G. In the following tables, the information needed to palpate each muscle is provided. The information includes position of the person, origin and insertion of the muscle, the line of pull of the muscle, the muscle's action, instructions to give to the person to make the muscle contract, and, finally, information on the best location to palpate the muscle.

Sitting Position

ANTERIOR DELTOID:	Located superficially and anterior to the shoulder joint (Fig. 9-12).
	FIGURE 9-12. Anterior deltoid.
Position of person:	Sitting facing the examiner with the arm relaxed at the side.
Origin:	Lateral third of the clavicle.
Insertion:	Deltoid tuberosity.
Line of pull:	When shoulder is abducted to 90°, line of pull is primarily horizontal. When shoulder is in anatomical position, line of pull is mostly vertical.
Muscle action:	Prime mover for horizontal adduction when the shoulder is abducted to 90°. In anatomical position, prime mover for flexion, abduction, and medial rotation.
Palpate:	Approximately 2 inches distal to the lateral clavicle.
Instructions to person:	Flex your shoulder to 90°. You can extend or flex your elbow.

(Continued...)

Sitting Position *(continued)*

MIDDLE DELTOID:	Located superficially and superior to the shoulder joint.

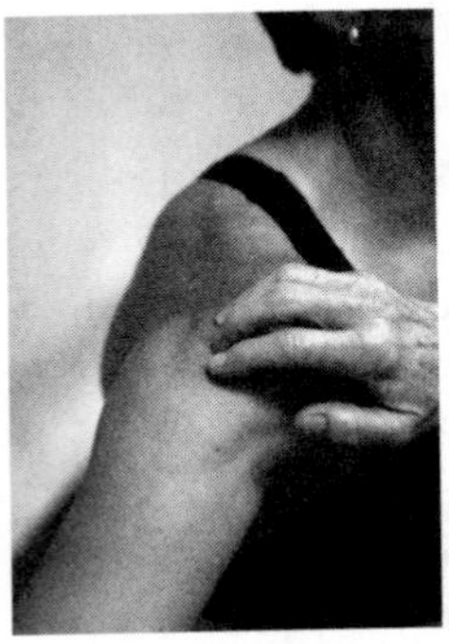

FIGURE 9-13. Middle deltoid.

Position of person:	Sitting facing the examiner with the arm relaxed at the side.
Origin:	Acromion process.
Insertion:	Deltoid tuberosity.
Line of pull:	Vertical.
Muscle action:	Prime mover for abduction.
Palpate:	Approximately 2 inches distal to the acromion process on the lateral aspect of the humerus.
Instructions to person:	Raise your arm out to the side to 90°. You can extend or flex your elbow.
SUPRASPINATUS:	Located deep to the upper trapezius.
Position of person:	Sitting facing away from the examiner with the arm relaxed at the side.
Origin:	Supraspinous fossa of the scapula.
Insertion:	Greater tubercle of the humerus.
Line of pull:	Horizontal.
Muscle action:	Prime mover for shoulder abduction. Contributes to stabilizing head of humerus in glenoid fossa.
Palpate:	This muscle is difficult to palpate because it is deep to the upper trapezius. The muscle belly is superior to the spine of the scapula in the supraspinatus fossa.
Instructions to person:	Raise your arm out to the side to 90°. You can extend or flex your elbow.

(Continued...)

CORACOBRACHIALIS:	Located deep to the anterior deltoid and the pectoralis major, and anterior to the shoulder joint.
	FIGURE 9-14. Palpating the origin of the coracobrachialis.
Position of person:	Sitting facing the examiner with the arm relaxed at the side.
Origin:	Coracoid process of the scapula.
Insertion:	Medial surface of the humerus near the midpoint of the shaft.
Line of pull:	Vertical.
Muscle action:	Stabilizes the shoulder and assists with flexion and adduction.
Palpate:	This muscle is difficult to palpate because it is deep to other shoulder muscles. Palpate origin on the coracoid process. A method to isolate the muscle is to place the person's hand on the hip and, while the person isometrically adducts the shoulder joint, palpate on the anterior medial surface of the proximal humerus.
Instructions to person:	Place your hand on your hip, pull your arm toward your body without letting it move. This is called an isometric contraction.

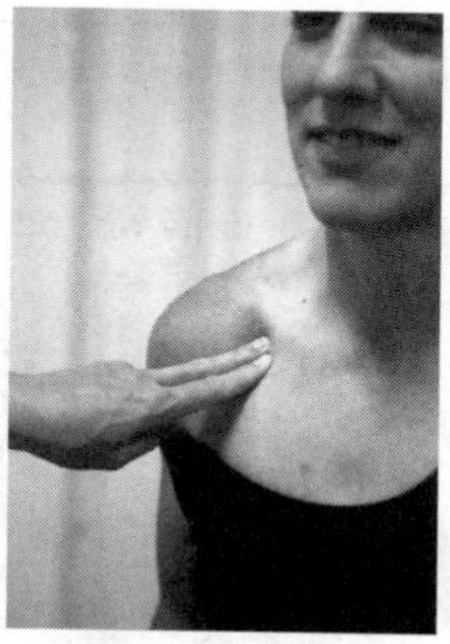

Prone Position

POSTERIOR DELTOID:	Located superficially and posterior to the shoulder joint.
	FIGURE 9-15. Palpating the posterior deltoid.
Position of person:	Lie prone with the shoulder abducted to 90° and the elbow flexed over the edge of the table.
Origin:	Spine of the scapula.
Insertion:	Deltoid tuberosity.
Line of pull:	Oblique. When shoulder is abducted to 90°, the line of pull is primarily horizontal.
Muscle action:	Shoulder abduction, extension, hyperextension, lateral rotation, and horizontal abduction.

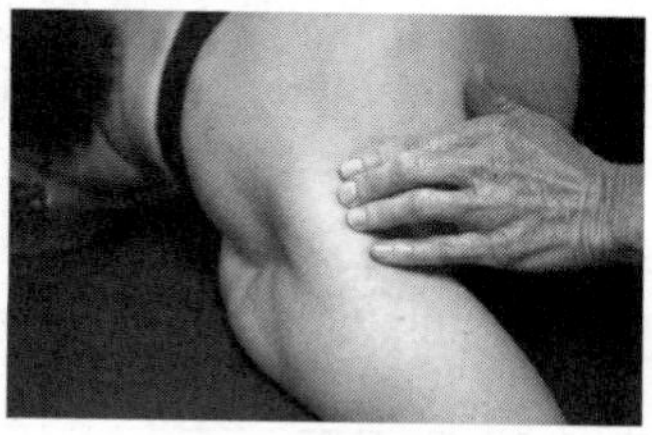

(Continued...)

Prone Position (continued)

Palpate:	On the posterior surface of the shoulder joint.
Instructions to person:	Lift your arm off the table by raising your elbow toward the ceiling.
LATISSIMUS DORSI:	Located superficially on the posterior thorax.

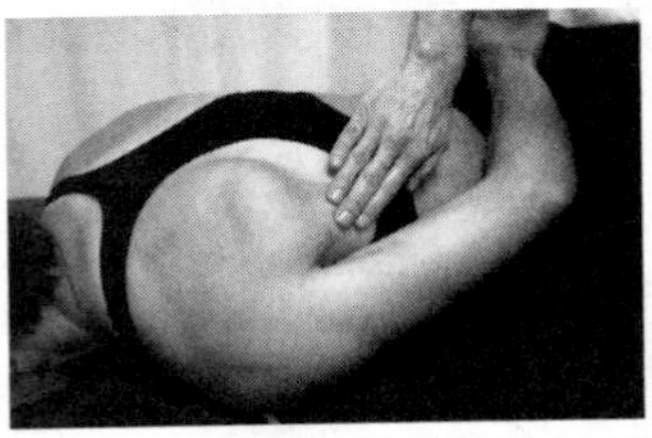

FIGURE 9-16. Palpating the latissimus dorsi.

Position of person:	Lie prone with the arm medially rotated at the side.
Origin:	Spinous process of T7–L5 via dorsolumbar fascia, posterior surface of the sacrum, iliac crest, and lower three ribs.
Insertion:	Medial lip of the bicipital groove of the humerus.
Line of pull:	Diagonal (mostly vertical).
Muscle action:	Prime mover for shoulder extension, hyperextension, medial rotation, and adduction. With the UE fixed, it lifts the pelvis.
Palpate:	On the side of the thorax near the axillae.
Instructions to person:	Place your hand on your low back and reach across your back toward your opposite hip.
TERES MAJOR:	Located superficially and posterior between the scapula and humerus.
Position of person:	Lie prone with the arm medially rotated at the side.
Origin:	Axillary border of the scapula near the inferior angle.
Insertion:	Crest of the humerus just inferior to the lesser tubercle and next to the insertion of the latissimus dorsi muscle.
Line of pull:	Diagonal.
Muscle action:	Prime mover for shoulder extension, medial rotation, and adduction.
Palpate:	On the lateral border of the scapula below the axillae.
Alternative method:	In the prone position, abduct the shoulder joint to 90° with the elbow flexed over the edge of the table so that the forearm is off the table and pronated. Medially rotate the shoulder joint by raising the palm of the hand toward the ceiling. Palpate the muscle belly lateral and superior to the inferior angle of the scapula.
Instructions to person:	Place your hand on your low back and reach across your back toward your opposite hip.

(Continued...)

INFRASPINATUS:	Located mostly superficially on the scapula with some parts deep to the middle and lower trapezius. **FIGURE 9-17.** Palpating the infraspinatus.
Position of person:	Lie prone with the shoulder at 90° of abduction and the elbow flexed over the edge of the table.
Origin:	Infraspinous fossa of scapula.
Insertion:	Greater tubercle of the humerus.
Line of pull:	Mostly horizontal.
Muscle action:	Prime mover for lateral rotation and horizontal abduction and assistive for extension.
Palpate:	Over the infraspinous fossa below the spine of the scapula.
Instructions to person:	Raise the back of your hand toward the ceiling.
TERES MINOR:	Located on the posterior scapula mostly superficial with some parts deep to the trapezius and deltoid. **FIGURE 9-18.** Palpating the teres minor.
Position of person:	Lie prone with the shoulder at 90° of abduction and the elbow flexed over the edge of the table.
Origin:	Axillary border of the scapula.
Insertion:	Greater tubercle of the humerus.
Line of pull:	Diagonal.
Muscle action:	Prime mover for lateral rotation and horizontal abduction.
Palpate:	Palpate origin along the axillary border of the scapula. Palpate muscle belly on posterior shoulder joint.
Instructions to person:	Raise your hand so the back of your hand is toward the ceiling.

Supine Position

SUBSCAPULARIS:	Located deep in the axillae.
Position of person:	Lie supine with the arm at the side and the elbow flexed to 90°.
Origin:	Anterior surface of the scapula in the subscapular fossa.

(Continued...)

Supine Position (continued)

Insertion:	Lesser tubercle of the humerus.
Line of pull:	Horizontal.
Muscle action:	Prime mover for medial rotation.
Palpate:	At the insertion, or in the axillae anterior to the latissimus dorsi.
Instructions to person:	Pull your hand to your abdomen while I resist the motion.
PECTORALIS MAJOR— CLAVICULAR PORTION:	Located superficially on the anterior thorax. 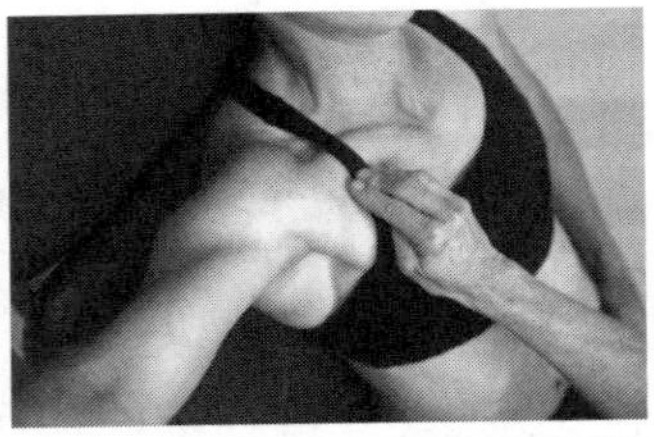 FIGURE 9-19. Palpating the pectoralis major clavicular portion.
Position of person:	Lie supine with the shoulder in 60° of abduction.
Origin:	Medial one-third of the clavicle.
Insertion:	Lateral lip of the bicipital groove of the humerus.
Line of pull:	Mostly vertical when the shoulder is in extension.
Muscle action:	Prime mover of flexion to 60°. With the sternal portion, it contributes to adduction, medial rotation, and horizontal adduction.
Palpate:	Just below the clavicle.
Instructions to person:	Raise your arm across your body toward the opposite shoulder.
PECTORALIS MAJOR— STERNAL PORTION:	Located superficially on the anterior thorax. 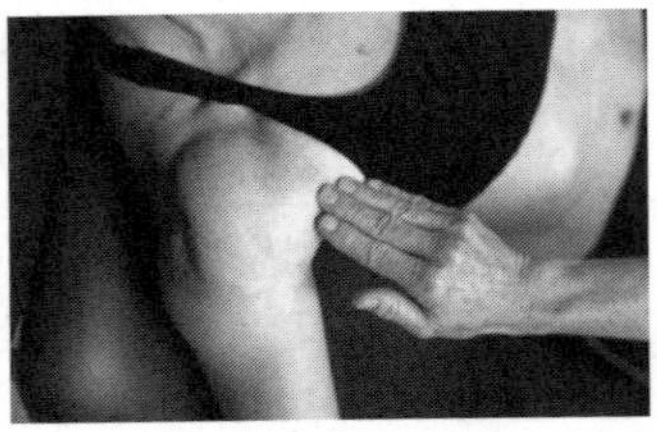 FIGURE 9-20. Palpating the pectoralis major sternal portion.
Position of person:	Lie supine with the shoulder in 120° of abduction.
Origin:	Sternum and costal cartilage of the first six ribs.
Insertion:	Lateral lip of the bicipital groove of the humerus.
Line of pull:	Mostly vertical when shoulder is in full flexion.
Muscle action:	Prime mover of shoulder extension against resistance—gravity or other force—from full flexion (180°) to about 120°. With the clavicular portion, it contributes to adduction, medial rotation, and horizontal adduction.
Palpate:	At the origin or at the lower anterior border of the axillae.
Instructions to person:	Move your arm across your body toward the opposite hip.

7. Use a disarticulated skeleton or anatomical model of the shoulder joint and apply the rules of joint arthrokinematics and the concave-convex rule to perform the following activities.

    A. The head of the humerus is _____ concave or _____ convex.

    The glenoid fossa is _____ concave or _____ convex.

    B. Move the distal bone, the humerus, on the proximal bone, the glenoid fossa of the scapula in all planes of motion. This is an open kinetic chain activity.

    C. Observe the movement of the head of the humerus on the glenoid fossa. Circle the motions that you observed.

    Spin   Roll   Glide   None

    D. Observe the movement of the distal end of the humerus in relation to the movement of the proximal end of the humerus as you move the head of the humerus on the

    glenoid fossa. Does the distal end of the humerus move in the _____ same or

    _____ opposite direction as the proximal end of the humerus?

    E. List the muscles that assist the head of the humerus to move in the glenoid fossa without impingement against the acromion.

    _____

    _____

8. Standing in the anatomical position and holding a backpack in one hand with the elbow extended.

    A. The force acting on the shoulder joint is _____ approximation or _____ traction.

    B. Name the muscles acting at the shoulder joint to counteract the force produced by the backpack.

    _____

    _____

    _____

    C. Name the muscles acting at the shoulder girdle to counteract the force produced by the backpack.

    _____

    _____

9. A person with zero strength of the elbow extensors can extend the elbow under specific conditions. In a long sitting position with arms laterally rotated and hands placed on the supporting surface slightly posterior and lateral to the trunk, the pectoralis major muscle can extend the elbow.

    A. Is this _____ an open or _____ a closed chain activity?

    B. Explain how the pectoralis major muscle extends the elbow in the position described.

    _____

    C. Can this be accomplished if the hand is not anchored? _____ Yes _____ No

10. Analyze what happens when an individual lying supine in the anatomical position raises both arms to 180° of flexion causing the lumbar lordosis to increase.

    A. What shoulder joint motion was performed?

    _____

    B. What muscle is being elongated simultaneously over more than one joint?

    _____

    C. Is this an example of active or passive insufficiency? _____

    D. Explain how this causes an increased lumbar lordosis:

    _____

    _____

11. Diagram the lever that describes abduction of the shoulder joint from 0° to 90° performed in the side-lying position.

    A. Draw a stick figure performing shoulder abduction in the side-lying position.

    B. Draw arrows to indicate the direction of the movement, the direction of the pull of the muscle, and the direction of gravity.

    C. Label the arrow that represents force with "F" and the arrow that represents resistance with "R."

12. Analyze the activity of shoulder abduction diagrammed in question 11 by answering the following questions:

    A. What is the "axis" of the motion? _____

    B. Is the movement with or against gravity? _____

    C. Is gravity or muscle the "force" producing the movement? _____

    D. Is gravity or muscle the "resistance" to the movement? _____

    E. Which major muscle group is the agonist? _____

    F. Which major muscle group is the antagonist? _____

    G. Is the agonist acting to overcome gravity or to slow down gravity? _____

    H. Is the agonist performing a concentric or an eccentric contraction? _____

    I. Is the antagonist contracting? _____

    J. Is this an open or closed kinetic chain activity? _____

13. Diagram the lever that describes *abduction of the shoulder joint* from 90° to 180° performed in the side-lying position.

    A. Draw a stick figure performing shoulder abduction from 90° to 180° in the side-lying position.

    B. Draw arrows to indicate the direction of the movement, the direction of the pull of the muscle, and the direction of gravity.

    C. Label the arrow that represents force with "F" and the arrow that represents resistance with "R."

14. Analyze the activity of shoulder abduction diagrammed in question 13 by answering the following questions:

    A. What is the "axis" of the motion? _____

    B. Is the movement with or against gravity? _____

    C. Is gravity or muscle the "force" producing the movement? _____

    D. Is gravity or muscle the "resistance" to the movement? _____

    E. Which major muscle group is the agonist? _____

    F. Which major muscle group is the antagonist? _____

    G. Is the agonist acting to overcome gravity or to slow down gravity? _____

    H. Is the agonist performing a concentric or an eccentric contraction? _____

    I. Is the antagonist contracting? _____

    J. Is this an open or closed kinetic chain activity? _____

15. Diagram the lever that describes *adduction of the shoulder joint* from 180° to 90° performed in the side-lying position.

    A. Draw a stick figure performing shoulder adduction in the side-lying position.

    B. Draw arrows to indicate the direction of the movement, the direction of the pull of the muscle, and the direction of gravity.

    C. Label the arrow that represents force with "F" and the arrow that represents resistance with "R."

16. Analyze the activity of shoulder adduction diagrammed in question 15 by answering the following questions:

    A. What is the "axis" of the motion? _____

    B. Is the movement with or against gravity? _____

    C. Is gravity or muscle the "force" producing the movement? _____

    D. Is gravity or muscle the "resistance" to the movement? _____

    E. Which major muscle group is the agonist? _____

    F. Which major muscle group is the antagonist? _____

    G. Is the agonist acting to overcome gravity or to slow down gravity? _____

    H. Is the agonist performing a concentric or an eccentric contraction? _____

    I. Is the antagonist contracting? _____

    J. Is this an open or closed kinetic chain activity? _____

17. Diagram the lever that describes *adduction of the shoulder joint* from 90° to 0° performed in the side-lying position.

    A. Draw a stick figure performing shoulder adduction from 90° to 0° in the side-lying position.

    B. Draw arrows to indicate the direction of the movement, the direction of the pull of the muscle, and the direction of gravity.

    C. Label the arrow that represents force with "F" and the arrow that represents resistance with "R."

18. Analyze the activity of shoulder adduction diagrammed in question 17 by answering the following questions:

    A. What is the "axis" of the motion? _____

    B. Is the movement with or against gravity? _____

    C. Is gravity or muscle the "force" producing the movement? _____

    D. Is gravity or muscle the "resistance" to the movement? _____

    E. Which major muscle group is the agonist? _____

    F. Which major muscle group is the antagonist? _____

    G. Is the agonist acting to overcome gravity or to slow down gravity? _____

    H. Is the agonist performing a concentric or an eccentric contraction? _____

    I. Is the antagonist contracting? _____

    J. Is this an open or closed kinetic chain activity? _____

■ ■ ■ Post-Lab Questions

Student's Name _____ Date Due _____

After you have completed the Worksheets and Lab Activities, answer the following questions without using your book or notes. When finished, check your answers.

1. When performing shoulder flexion in an open kinetic chain, is the concave surface moving on the convex surface or is the convex surface moving on the concave surface?

   _____

   _____

2. List the muscles of the shoulder joint that attach on the greater tubercle of the humerus.

   _____

   _____

3. List the muscles that cross the shoulder joint posteriorly.

   _____

   _____

4. List the motions of the shoulder joint.

   _____

   _____

5. You are to treat a house painter who fell off a ladder. In addition to sustaining an anterior dislocation of the shoulder, he has axillary nerve damage. Which muscle(s) may be weakened because of the nerve injury?

   _____

6. You are palpating the coracoid process and thinking about the muscle(s) attached to it. List the shoulder joint muscle(s) attaching to the coracoid process.

   _____

   _____

7. You are palpating the bicipital groove and thinking about the muscles attached on either side.

   A. List the muscle(s) attached to the lateral side of the bicipital groove:

   _____

   B. List the muscle(s) attached to the medial side of the bicipital groove:

   _____

8. A. The teres major and minor muscles attach along the _____ border of the scapula.

   B. The teres _____ muscle is located superior to the teres _____ muscle along the scapular border identified in A.

   C. The teres _____ muscle remains on the posterior surface of the shoulder while the teres _____ muscle crosses to the anterior surface.

   D. The _____ muscle, running vertically, passes between the teres major and minor in the axilla.

9. The rotator cuff muscles insert deep to the _____ muscle.

10. The _____ and the _____ muscles are responsible for shoulder hyperextension.

11. The _____ muscle is inferior to the supraspinatus muscle, superior to the teres minor and, in part, deep to the trapezius and deltoid muscles.

12. While palpating the borders of the axilla, you are thinking that the anterior border is formed by the _____ muscle and the posterior border is formed by the _____ muscle.

13. While palpating the acromion process, you are thinking that the _____ muscle passes inferior to the acromion process.

14. The nerve that innervates the deltoid muscle is often injured when the shoulder dislocates.
    A. Identify the nerve.

    _____

    B. Describe the sensory area innervated by this nerve.

    _____

    _____

15. Glenohumeral muscles are often referred to as SIT, SITS, and rotator cuff muscles. Indicate in the following table, if a muscle is a SIT, SITS, or rotator cuff muscle.

Muscles	SIT	SITS	Rotator Cuff
Subscapularis			
Supraspinatus			
Infraspinatus			
Teres minor			

Chapter 10

Elbow Joint

Worksheets

Student's Name ______________________ Date Due ______________

Complete the following questions prior to lab class.

1. Define the following term:

   Carrying angle: ______________________

2. On Figures 10-1 through 10-4, label the following bones and landmarks:

   SCAPULA: Infraglenoid tubercle Supraglenoid tubercle

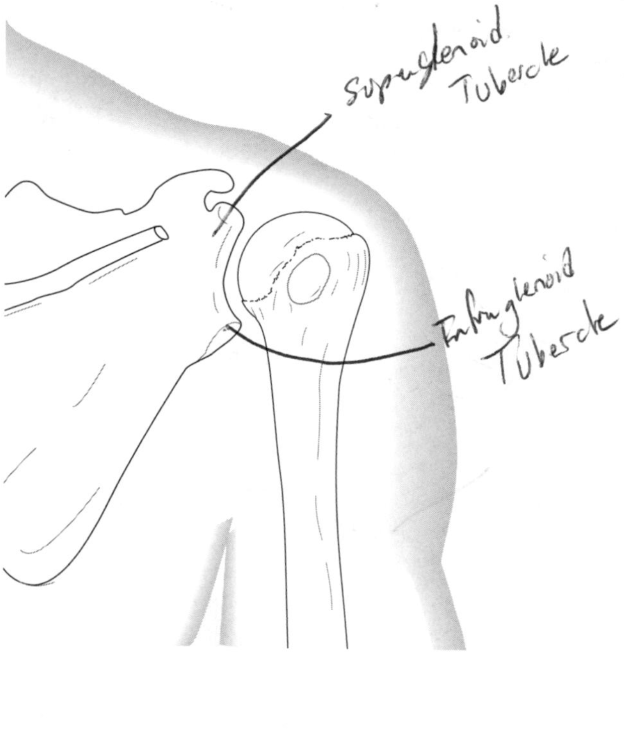

FIGURE 10-1. Landmarks of the scapula, posterior view (acromion has been removed).

HUMERUS: Trochlea   Capitulum   Medial epicondyle
Lateral epicondyle   Lateral supracondylar ridge
Olecranon fossa

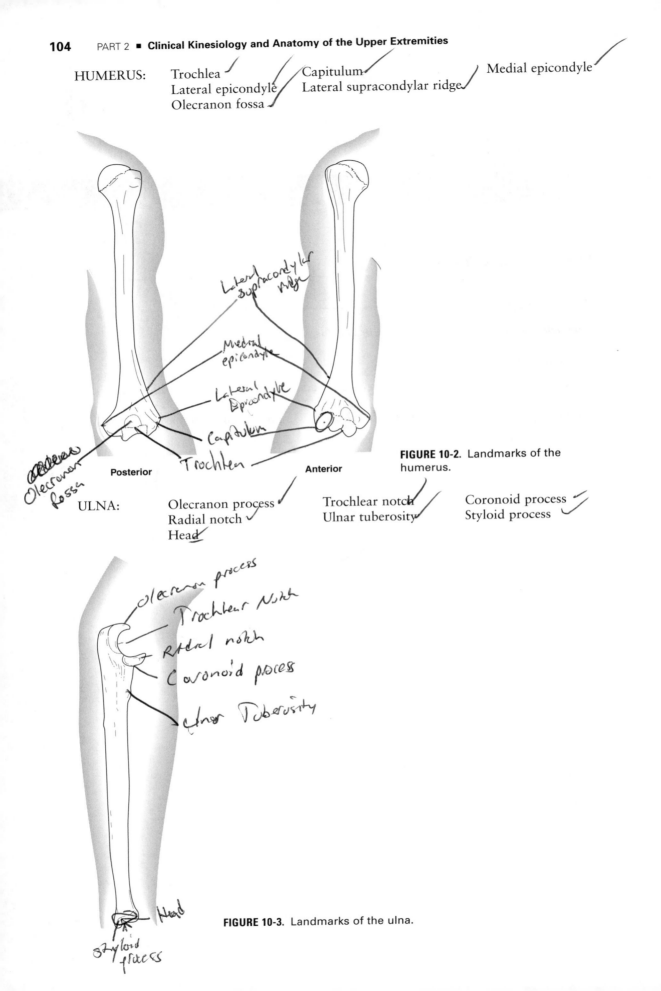

FIGURE 10-2. Landmarks of the humerus.

ULNA: Olecranon process   Trochlear notch   Coronoid process
Radial notch   Ulnar tuberosity   Styloid process
Head

FIGURE 10-3. Landmarks of the ulna.

RADIUS: Head   Radial tuberosity   Styloid process

Hed

Radial Tuberosity

Styloid process

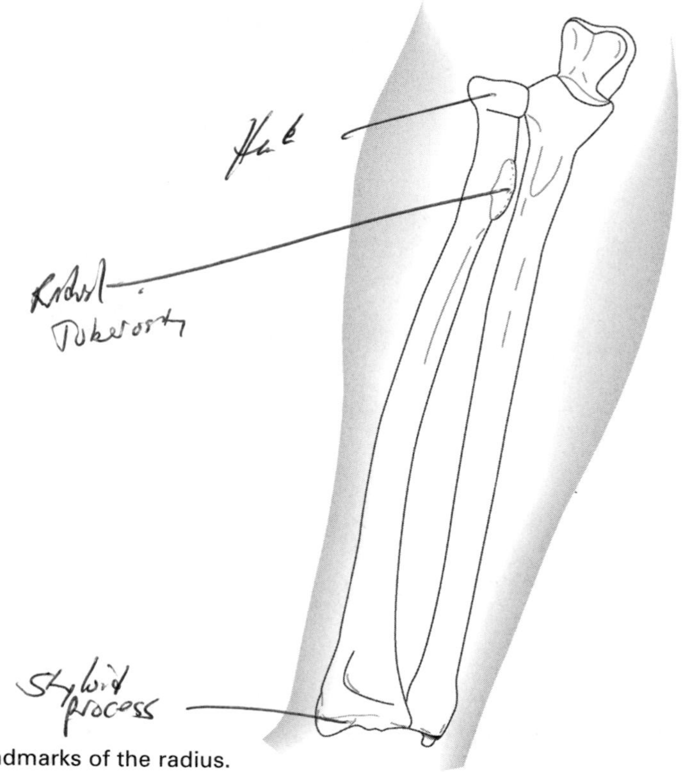

FIGURE 10-4. Landmarks of the radius.

3. On the Figures 10-5 and 10-6:
   A. Label the joints and bones
      Humerus   Ulna   Radius
      Elbow joint ✓   Proximal radioulnar joint

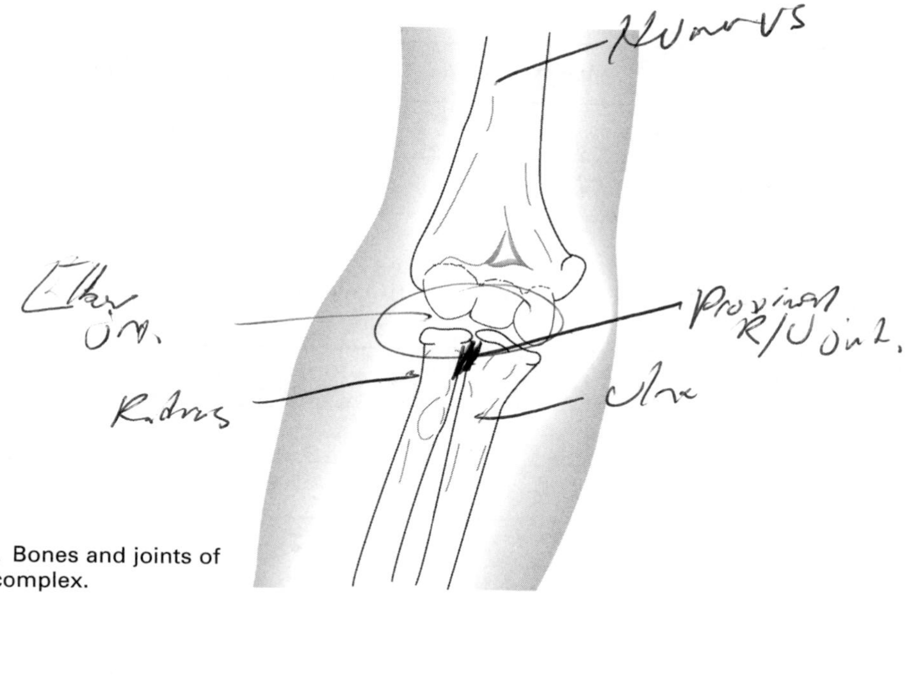

Humerus

Elbow Jn.

Radius

Proximal R/U Jnt.

Ulna

FIGURE 10-5. Bones and joints of the elbow complex.

B. Label the following structures:

Medial collateral ligament
Annular ligament
Capsule

Lateral collateral ligament
Interosseous membrane
Radius

Ulna

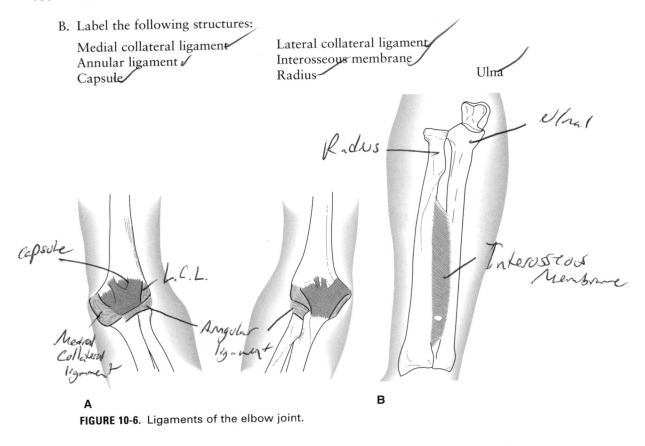

FIGURE 10-6. Ligaments of the elbow joint.

4. Are the motions available at the proximal and distal radioulnar joints the _____ same

   or _____different?

5. For the following joints, identify the shape of the joint, the degrees of freedom, motions, plane, and axis.

Joint	Shape of Joint	Degrees of Freedom	Motions	Plane	Axis
Elbow					
Radioulnar					

6. At each of the following joints, identify which surface is concave and which is convex.

Joint	Concave	Convex
Elbow		
Radioulnar		

7. On Figures 10-7 through 10-10:

   A. Label the origin and insertion of the muscles listed.
      Color the origin in red and the insertion in blue.

   B. Join the origin and insertion to show the line of pull.

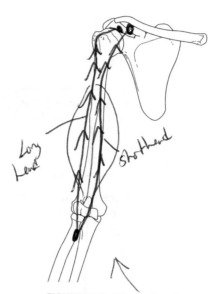

FIGURE 10-7. Biceps brachii.

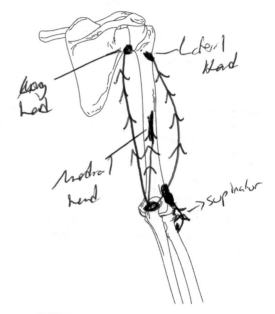

FIGURE 10-8. Triceps brachii and supinator.

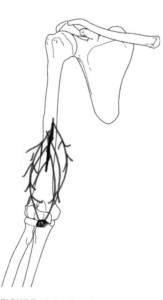

FIGURE 10-9. Brachialis.

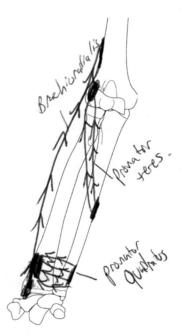

FIGURE 10-10. Brachioradialis, pronator teres, and pronator quadratus.

8. For each of the joints below provide the close-packed position and the loose-packed position. (Refer to Chapter 4.)

Joint	Close-Packed	Loose-Packed
Elbow		
Radioulnar		

9. For each of the following joints, describe the end feel. (Refer to Chapter 4.)

Joint	Bony	Capsular	Soft Tissue Approximation
Elbow			
Radioulnar			

10. Match each ligament and structure to the appropriate function or characteristic. Some answers may be used more than once. Some functions or characteristics may have more than one answer.

_____ Attaches to humeral epicondyle and lateral side of ulna

_____ Is triangular in shape

_____ Is ring-shaped

_____ Keeps lateral side of joint from separating when stressed

_____ Keeps medial side of joint from separating when stressed

_____ Keeps radius and ulna in contact

_____ Strengthens joint capsule

_____ Attaches to humerus, radius, and ulna

A. Medial collateral ligament

B. Lateral collateral ligament

C. Annular ligament

D. Interosseous membrane

E. Joint capsule

■ ■ ■ Lab Activities

Student's Name _____ Date Due _____

1. Perform motions of the elbow and forearm joints with your partner.
   A. Perform a motion and then your partner names the motion you performed.
   B. Your partner states a motion and then you perform that motion.

2. Using the worksheets question 5 for reference, for each of the motions available at the elbow and radioulnar joints:
   A. Place your open left hand in the correct orientation to represent the plane of a motion.
   B. Place your right index finger to indicate the axis of that motion.

3. Observe the amount of motion available at each joint in each plane.

   For each of the motions available at the elbow and radioulnar joints, estimate the degrees of motion available by checking the box that *most closely* describes that amount of motion. (Do not measure with a goniometer.)

Motions	0°–45°	46°–90°	91°–135°	136°–180°
Elbow				
Radioulnar				

4. Passively move your partner's elbow through the available range of motion noting the end feel. If possible repeat with several people. Review question 9 in the worksheets for the normal end feel.

   A. Is your partner's end feel consistent with normal end feel?

   _____

   B. What structures create the end feel for this joint?

   _____

5. On the skeleton, anatomical models, and at least one partner, locate, palpate, and observe the following structures. The reference position is the anatomical position. Having pictures for reference is helpful when trying to find structures. Not all structures are palpable on your partner.

Scapula

Infraglenoid tubercle	The raised portion on the inferior lip of the glenoid fossa; provides attachment of the long head of the triceps muscle. It is located deep in joint and cannot be palpated.
Supraglenoid tubercle	The raised portion on the superior lip of the glenoid fossa; provides attachment for the long head of the biceps brachii muscle. It is located deep to the acromion process and cannot be palpated.
Coracoid process	The projection on the anterior surface, provides attachment for the short head of the biceps brachii. Palpate on the proximal anteriolateral chest wall under the clavicle. Deep to the pectoralis major muscle, the coracoid process can be palpated by pressing deeply into the tissue. This may be uncomfortable for the person being palpated.

Humerus

Trochlea	Located at the medial side of the distal end; articulates with the ulna. This structure is within the joint and thus cannot be palpated.
Capitulum	Located on the lateral side of the distal end next to the trochlea; articulates with the head of the radius. This structure is within the joint and thus cannot be palpated.
Medial epicondyle	Palpate on the medial side of the distal end of the humerus above the trochlea; larger and more prominent than the lateral epicondyle; it provides attachment for the pronator teres muscles. **FIGURE 10-11.** Palpating the medial epicondyle.
Lateral epicondyle	Can be observed and palpated on the lateral side of the distal end of the humerus above the capitulum; provides attachment for the anconeus and supinator muscles. **FIGURE 10-12.** Palpating the lateral epicondyle.
Lateral supracondylar ridge	Palpate above the lateral epicondyle; provides attachment for the brachioradialis muscle. **FIGURE 10-13.** Palpating the lateral supracondylar ridge.

(*Continued...*)

Olecranon fossa	Located on the posterior distal surface of the humerus between the medial and lateral epicondyles; articulates with the olecranon process of the ulna. Because it is deep to the triceps and olecranon process, it can be difficult to palpate. Flexing the elbow to about 90° moves the olecranon process out of the fossa without causing the triceps to become taut. This may allow the fossa to be palpated just above the olecranon process posteriorly. 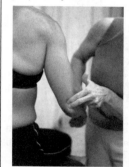 **FIGURE 10-14.** Palpating the olecranon fossa.

Ulna

Olecranon process	Large prominent point of the elbow posteriorly. Palpate on the posterior proximal end of the ulna; forms the prominent point of the elbow and provides attachment for the triceps muscle. **FIGURE 10-15.** Palpating the olecranon process.
Trochlear notch	Located on the anterior surface of the proximal end; articulates with the trochlea of the humerus. This structure is located within the joint and thus cannot be palpated.
Coronoid process	Located on the anterior surface of the proximal end distal to the trochlear notch; provides attachment for the brachialis muscle. Located deep to muscles. Cannot be palpated.
Radial notch	Located on the proximal end of the lateral side just distal to the trochlear notch; articulation point for the head of the radius. Located deep to muscles. Cannot be palpated.
Ulnar tuberosity	Below the coronoid process; provides attachment for the brachialis muscle. Located deep to muscles. Cannot be palpated.

(Continued...)

Ulna *(continued)*

Styloid process	Palpate on the distal end on the posterior medial surface. 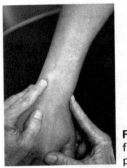 **FIGURE 10-16.** The examiner's left index finger is palpating the ulnar styloid process.
Head	The distal end; the ulnar notch of the radius pivots around it during pronation and supination. Cannot be palpated.

Radius

Head	Palpate on the proximal lateral aspect of the radius; articulates with the capitulum of the humerus. Hold your partner's forearm flexed at the elbow. Place the fingers of your other hand on the lateral aspect of the forearm just distal to the elbow joint. You should feel the head move under your fingers as you pronate and supinate the forearm. **FIGURE 10-17.** Palpating the head of the radius.
Radial tuberosity	Located distal to the head on the medial side near the proximal end; provides attachment for the biceps brachii muscle. Located deep to muscles and cannot be palpated.
Styloid process	Palpate on the posterior lateral side of the distal end of the radius; provides attachment for the brachioradialis muscle. Not as prominent as the ulnar styloid process. **FIGURE 10-18.** The examiner's right index finger is palpating the radial styloid process.

Ligaments/Structures

Medial collateral ligament	Palpate on the medial side of the elbow; attaches on the medial epicondyle of the humerus and the coronoid process and olecranon process of the ulna.
Lateral collateral ligament	Palpate on the lateral side of the elbow; attaches on the lateral epicondyle of the humerus, the annular ligament, and the lateral side of the ulna.
Annular ligament	Encircles the head of the radius; attaches anteriorly and posteriorly to the radial notch of the ulna. Located deep to muscles and cannot be palpated.
Interosseous membrane	Between the radius and ulna. Located deep to muscles and thus cannot be palpated.

6. Use a disarticulated skeleton or anatomical model of the elbow joint and apply the rules of joint arthrokinematics and the concave-convex rule to perform the following activities.

   A. Underline the correct answer.

The ulna is:	Concave	Convex
The radius is:	Concave	Convex
The medial surface of the distal humerus is:	Concave	Convex
The lateral surface of the distal humerus is:	Concave	Convex

   B. Move the distal bones, the radius and ulna, on the proximal bone, the humerus, in all planes of motion.

   C. Observe the movement of the distal bones, the radius and ulna, on the proximal bone, the humerus. Circle the motions that you observed.

   Roll   Spin   Glide

   D. Observe the movement of the distal ends of the radius and ulna in relation to the movement of the proximal end of the radius and ulna as you move the bones on the

   humerus. Do the distal ends of the radius and ulna move in the _____ same or

   _____ opposite direction as the proximal ends of the radius and ulna?

   E. Move the proximal bone, the humerus of the elbow joint on the distal bones, the radius and ulna, as would occur in a closed kinetic chain activity.

   F. Observe the movement of the distal end of the humerus on the radius and ulna during a closed kinetic chain activity. Circle the motions you observe.

   Roll   Spin   Glide

   G. Observe the movement of the proximal end of the humerus. Does the distal end move

   in the _____ same or _____ opposite direction as the proximal end of the humerus during movement at the elbow joint in a closed kinetic chain activity?

7. Locate the following on the skeleton, anatomical models, and at least one partner:

   A. Locate the origin and insertion of the muscle on the skeleton.

   B. Stretch a large rubber band taut by placing one end at the origin and the other end at the insertion of a muscle on the skeleton.

   C. Perform the motion that the muscle does and observe how the rubber band becomes less taut and shorter, similar to the muscle shortening as it contracts.

D. Perform the opposite motion and observe how the rubber band becomes more taut and longer, similar to the muscle lengthening as it is being stretched.

E. After locating the muscle on the skeleton, locate the muscle on your partner. The position described for locating the muscle on your partner is the manual muscle test position for a fair or better grade of muscle strength. Not all origins, insertions, and muscle bellies can be palpated on your partner.

F. When possible, palpate the origin, insertion, and muscle belly of each muscle by:

1) Placing your fingers on the origin and insertion, and asking your partner to contract the muscle.

2) Moving your fingers from the origin and insertion over the contracting muscle.

3) Asking your partner to relax the muscle and again moving your fingers from the origin to the insertion over the muscle.

4) Note the difference between the contracting and relaxed muscle.

G. In the following tables, the information needed to palpate each muscle is provided. The information includes position of the person, origin and insertion of the muscle, the line of pull of the muscle, the muscle's action, instructions to give to the person to make the muscle contract, and, finally, information on the best location to palpate the muscle.

Sitting Position

BRACHIALIS:	Located on the anterior surface of the arm deep to the biceps brachii.
	FIGURE 10-19. Palpating the brachialis muscle.
Position of person:	Sit facing the examiner with the arm at the side and the forearm supinated.
Origin:	Anterior surface of the distal half of the humerus.
Insertion:	Coronoid process and ulna tuberosity of the ulna.
Line of pull:	Vertical on the anterior surface.
Muscle action:	Flexes the elbow.
Palpate:	Press your fingers deep on either side of the biceps tendon at the distal end of the humerus.
Instructions to person:	Keeping your palm up, bend your elbow.

(Continued...)

BRACHIORADIALIS:	Located superficially on the lateral aspect of the forearm.

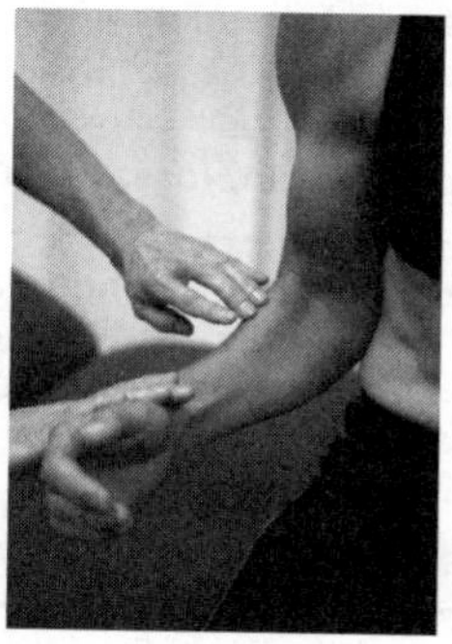

FIGURE 10-20. Palpating the brachioradialis muscle.

Position of person:	Sit facing the examiner with the arm at the side and the forearm in the midposition, halfway between supination and pronation.
Origin:	Lateral supracondylar ridge of the humerus.
Insertion:	Distal lateral aspect of the radius just proximal to the radial styloid process.
Line of pull:	Vertical on the anterior surface.
Muscle action:	Flexes the elbow.
Palpate:	Just distal to the elbow joint on the lateral side over the muscle belly.
Instructions to person:	Keeping the thumb up, bend your elbow.
BICEPS BRACHII:	Located superficially on the anterior aspect of the humerus.

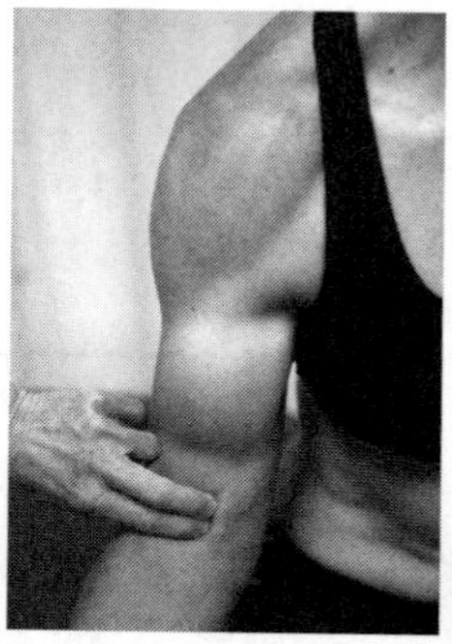

FIGURE 10-21. Palpating the distal tendon of the biceps brachii.

Position of person:	Sit facing the examiner with the arm at the side and the forearm supinated.
Origin:	Long head: Supraglenoid tubercle of the scapula. Short head: Coracoid process of the scapula.
Insertion:	Radial tuberosity of the radius.

(Continued...)

Sitting Position *(continued)*

Line of pull:	Vertical at the elbow joint and diagonal at the proximal radioulnar joint.
Muscle action:	Elbow flexion, forearm supination.
Palpate:	The origin of the long head cannot be palpated at its origin but can be palpated in the bicipital groove. The origin of the short head can be palpated just below the coracoid process.
Instructions to person:	Keeping your palm up, bend your elbow.
SUPINATOR:	Located deep on the lateral aspect of the elbow.

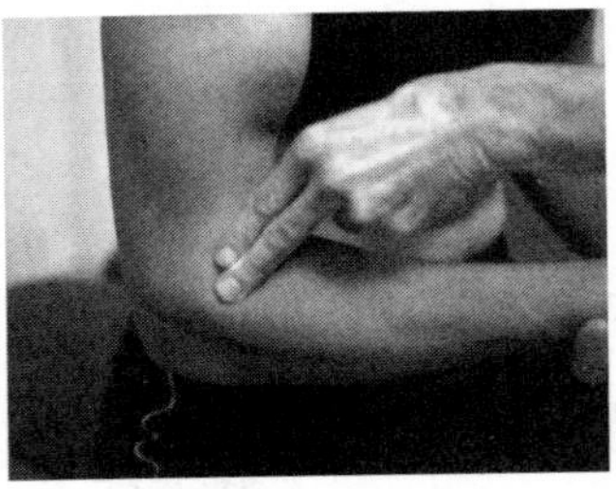

FIGURE 10-22. Palpating the supinator.

Position of person:	Sit facing the examiner with the arm at the side and the forearm in the midposition.
Origin:	Lateral epicondyle of the humerus and posterior lateral aspect of the adjacent ulna.
Insertion:	Anterior surface of the proximal radius.
Line of pull:	Diagonal and posterior to the joint.
Muscle action:	Supinates the forearm.
Palpate:	On the lateral aspect of the elbow.
Instructions to person:	Turn your palm up.
PRONATOR TERES:	Located superficially on the medial aspect of the elbow.

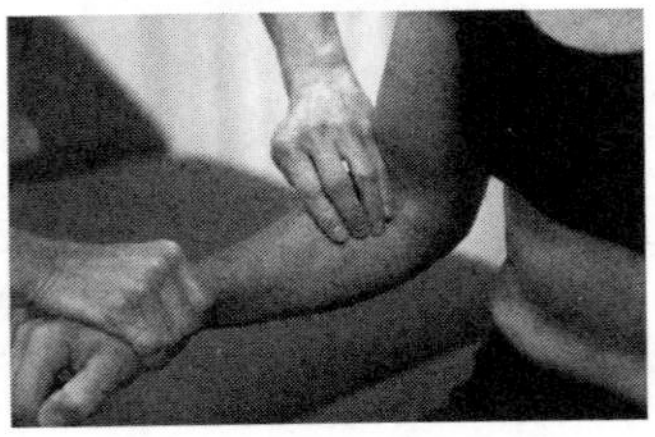

FIGURE 10-23. Palpating the pronator teres.

Position of person:	Sit with the arm at the side, the elbow flexed to 90°, and the forearm in the midposition.
Origin:	Medial epicondyle of the humerus and coronoid process of the ulna.
Insertion:	Lateral aspect of the radius at the midpoint of the shaft.
Line of pull:	Diagonal and anterior to the joint.

(Continued...)

Muscle action:	Pronates the forearm—turns the palm down.
Palpate:	On the anterior surface of the proximal third of the forearm between the origin and insertion. Resisting the pronation may make the muscle easier to find.
Instructions to person:	Turn your palm down.
PRONATOR QUADRATUS:	Located deep on the anterior distal surface of the forearm.
Position of person:	Sit with the arm at side, the elbow flexed to 90°, and the forearm in the midposition.
Origin:	Anterior surface of the distal quarter of the ulna.
Insertion:	Anterior surface of the distal quarter of the radius.
Line of pull:	Horizontal on the anterior surface.
Muscle action:	Pronates the forearm—turns the palm down.
Palpate:	The pronator quadratus may be difficult to palpate because it is deep to many tendons of the wrist and hand muscles.
Instructions to person:	Turn your palm down.

Prone Position

TRICEPS BRACHII:	Located superficially on the posterior surface of the humerus.
Position of person:	Lie prone with the shoulder abducted to 90° and the elbow flexed over the edge of the table. 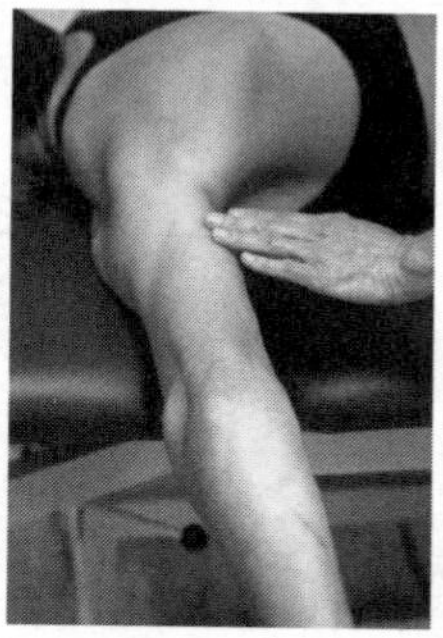 **FIGURE 10-24.** Palpating the triceps brachii.
Origin:	Long head: Infraglenoid tubercle of the scapula. Lateral head: Inferior to the greater tubercle on the posterior side of the humerus. Medial head: Posterior surface of the humerus.
Insertion:	Olecranon process of the ulna.
Line of pull:	Vertical on the posterior surface.
Muscle action:	Extends the elbow.

(Continued...)

Prone Position (continued)

Palpation:	Palpate the posterior surface of the humerus.
Instructions to person:	Raise your hand toward the ceiling.
ANCONEUS:	Located superficially on the posterior aspect of the elbow.
Position of person:	Lie prone with the shoulder abducted to 90° and the elbow flexed over the edge of the table.
Origin:	Lateral epicondyle of the humerus.
Insertion:	Lateral and inferior to the triceps on the olecranon process of the ulna.
Line of pull:	Diagonal and posterior to the joint.
Muscle action:	Assists in extending the elbow.
Palpation:	This small muscle is not present in all individuals and is difficult to separate from the triceps.
Instructions to person:	Raise your hand toward the ceiling.

8. The strength of a muscle can be tested with the individual in the test position for a fair grade or better. To test the strength of the elbow flexors in sitting, a person flexes his or her elbow to about 90° and holds that position as you try to move it into extension.

   To test the strength of the elbow extensors, a person lies prone with the shoulder abducted to 90° and the elbow flexed over the edge of the table. The person extends the elbow and holds that position as you try to move it into flexion.

   A. Test the strength of your partner's elbow flexors with the forearm positioned first in pronation, second in midposition, and third in supination.

   Did the position of the forearm affect the strength of the elbow flexors?

   _____

   Explain your answer.

   _____

   _____

   B. Test the strength of your partner's elbow extensors with the forearm positioned first in pronation, second in midposition, and third in supination.

   Did the position of the forearm affect the strength of the elbow extensors?

   _____

   Explain your answer.

   _____

   _____

9. Diagram the lever that describes the activity at the elbow joint as you perform a push-up from the prone position. Analyze the *down* motion.

   A. Draw a stick figure performing the push-up.

   B. Draw arrows to indicate the direction of the movement, the direction of the pull of the muscle, and the direction of gravity.

   C. Label the arrow that represents force with an "F" and the arrow that represents resistance with an "R."

10. Analyze the activity of the lowering motion of a push-up diagrammed in question 9 by answering the following questions:

    A. The starting range of motion is _____°, and the ending range of motion is _____°.

    B. What is the "axis" of the motion? _____

    C. Is the movement with or against gravity? _____

    D. Is gravity or muscle the "force" producing the movement? _____

    E. Is gravity or muscle the "resistance" to the movement? _____

    F. Which major muscle group is the agonist? _____

    G. Which major muscle group is the antagonist? _____

    H. Is the agonist acting to overcome gravity or to slow down gravity? _____

    I. Is the agonist performing a concentric or an eccentric contraction? _____

    J. Is the antagonist contracting? _____

    K. Is this an open or closed kinetic chain activity? _____

    L. In the full push-up position, is _____ traction or _____ approximation occurring at the elbow joint?

■ ■ ■ Post-Lab Questions

Student's Name _____ Date Due _____

After you have completed the Worksheets and Lab Activities, answer the following questions without using your book or notes. When finished, check your answers.

1. Name the ring-shaped ligament within which the radius rotates:

   _____

2. You are palpating the arm of a person who has had an anterior dislocation of the elbow.
   A. Name the muscle that lies deep to the biceps brachii near the distal end of the humerus.

   _____

   B. Name the muscle that lies deep to the biceps brachii at the shoulder.

   _____

3. Name the nerve that lies in the groove between the medial epicondyle and the olecranon

   process. _____

4. Match the nerve with the muscle it innervates—nerves may be used more than once.

   _____ Biceps brachii   A. Musculocutaneous

   _____ Triceps brachii   B. Radial

   _____ Pronator teres   C. Median

   _____ Pronator quadratus

   _____ Supinator

   _____ Brachialis

   _____ Brachioradialis

5. Which elbow flexors attach to the:

   Radius: _____

   Ulna: _____

6. Which elbow flexors attach to the humerus?

   _____

7. For each of the motions of the elbow and forearm listed check the muscle(s) that are the major contributes to the motion.

Motions	Brachialis	Brachioradialis	Biceps Brachii	Supinator	Triceps Brachii	Pronator Teres	Pronator Quadratus
Flexion							
Extension							
Supination							
Pronation							

8. List the joint positions that create passive insufficiency of
   A. Triceps brachii:

   _____

   _____

   B. Biceps brachii:

   _____

   _____

9. List the joint positions that create active insufficiency of:
   A. Triceps brachii:

   _____

   _____

   B. Biceps brachii:

   _____

   _____

10. Identify the following nonmuscular structures:
    A. This structure crosses the elbow vertically on the radial side attaching to the humerus and ulna: _____

    B. This structure crosses the elbow vertically on the ulnar side attaching to the humerus and ulna: _____

    C. This structure attaches only to the ulna: _____

    D. This structure connects the ulna and the radius via a broad attachment:

    _____

11. In the following activities, determine if the distal attachment is moving toward the proximal attachment or if the proximal attachment moving toward the distal attachment.

Activity	Proximal to Distal	Distal to Proximal
An individual pulls on a rope to bring a boat to shore.		
An individual climbs up a rope.		

Which of the above activities is an example of a reversal of muscle action?

_____

12. A person has had a midshift fracture of the humerus. A complication of this injury was damage to the radial nerve resulting in muscle paralysis.
    A. Which elbow and/or forearm muscles will have lost innervation?

       _____

       _____

    B. What motion(s) will the person have difficulty performing?

       _____

13. Which muscle lies deep to the wrist and finger flexors at the distal forearm?

    _____

14. Why must a muscle attach on the radius to be able to pronate or supinate the forearm?

    _____

15. A. Which elbow joint muscles do not attach to the radius?

       _____

    B. Do any of these muscles cause pronation or supination? _____ Yes _____ No

16. When elbow flexion without supination is desired, which muscle(s) prevents supination?

    _____

Chapter 11

Wrist

Worksheets

Student's Name ____________________ Date Due ____________

Complete the following questions prior to the lab class.

1. On the Figures 11-1 and 11-2:
   A. Label the following joints:
      Radiocarpal joint Midcarpal joint Carpometacarpal joint

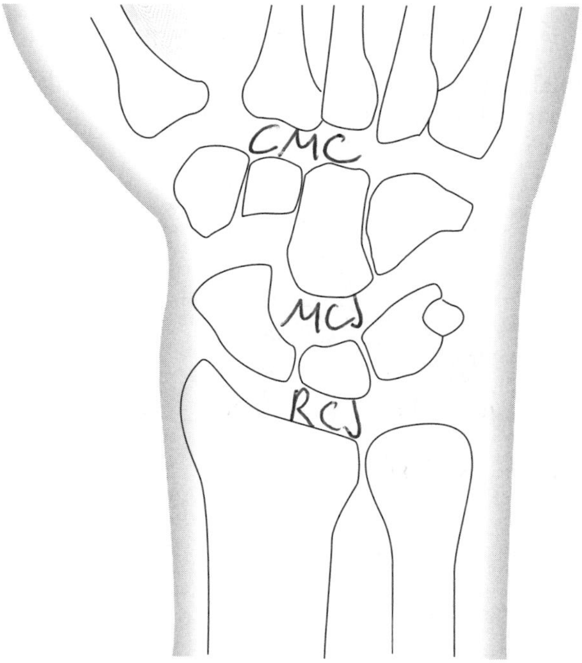

FIGURE 11-1. Joints of the wrist.

B. Label the following bones and landmarks:

Scaphoid   Lunate   Triquetrum
Pisiform   Capitate   Hamate
Trapezium   Trapezoid   Radial styloid process
Radius   Ulna   Articular disk
Metacarpals (1–5)

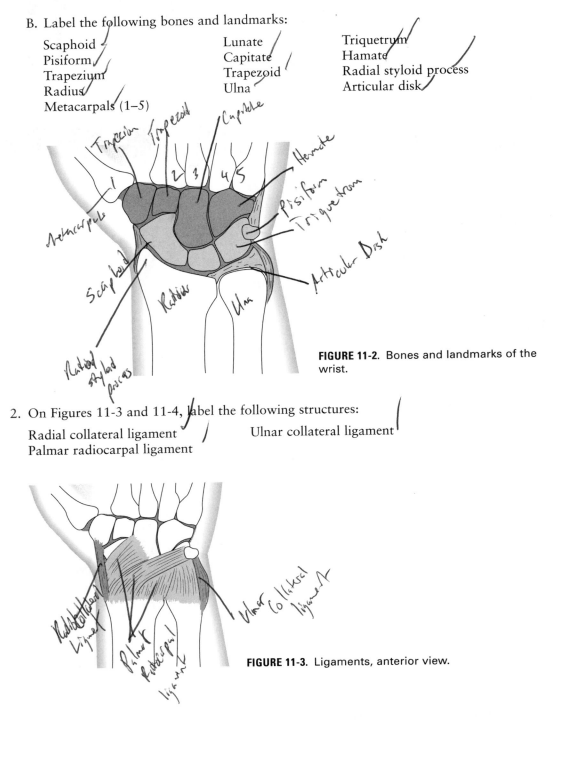

FIGURE 11-2. Bones and landmarks of the wrist.

2. On Figures 11-3 and 11-4, label the following structures:

Radial collateral ligament   Ulnar collateral ligament
Palmar radiocarpal ligament

FIGURE 11-3. Ligaments, anterior view.

Dorsal radiocarpal ligament
Radial collateral ligament

Ulnar styloid process
Ulnar collateral ligament

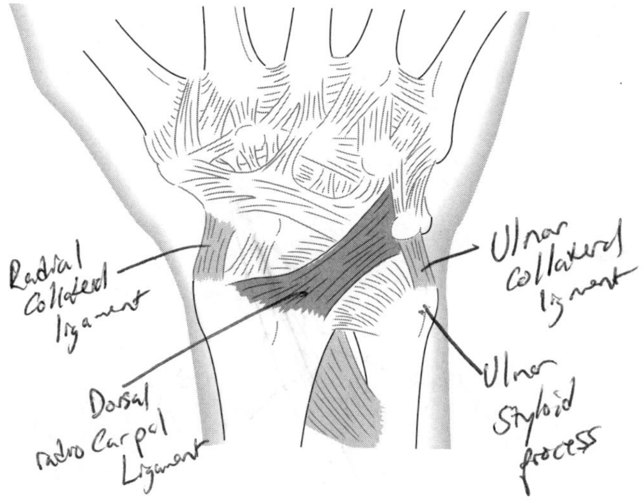

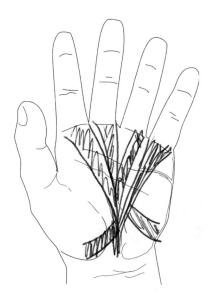

FIGURE 11-4. Ligaments, posterior view.

3. Draw in the palmar fascia on Figure 11-5.

FIGURE 11-5. Palmar fascia.

4. On Figures 11-6 and 11-7:

  A. Label the origin and insertion of the muscles shown.

     Color the origin in red and the insertion in blue.

  B. Join the origin and insertion to show the direction of the muscle fibers.

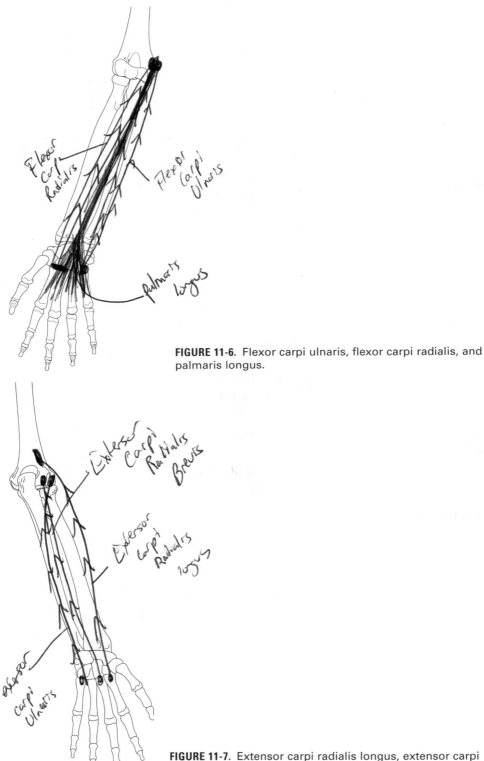

FIGURE 11-6. Flexor carpi ulnaris, flexor carpi radialis, and palmaris longus.

FIGURE 11-7. Extensor carpi radialis longus, extensor carpi radialis brevis, and extensor carpi ulnaris.

5. Match each function or characteristic with the appropriate structure. Use each term only once.

   _____ Limits extension   A. Radial collateral ligament

   _____ Filler between ulna and adjacent carpals   B. Ulnar collateral ligament

   _____ Provides lateral support   C. Palmar radiocarpal ligament

   _____ Limits flexion   D. Dorsal radiocarpal ligament

   _____ Provides protection and muscle attachment   E. Articular disk

   _____ Provides medial support   F. Palmar fascia

6. For the following joints, identify the type and number of planes of motion available.

Joint	Shape	Degrees of Freedom	Motions	Planes	Axis
Radiocarpal					
Midcarpal					

7. For the radiocarpal joint, identify which surface is concave and which is convex.

   Concave: _____

   Convex: _____

8. For the radiocarpal joint, provide the close-packed position and the loose-packed position. (Refer to Chapter 4.)

Joint	Close-Packed	Loose-Packed
Radiocarpal		

9. The end feel of a normal radiocarpal joint: (Refer to Chapter 4 for descriptions.)

   Flexion/extension

   _____ Bony   _____ Capsular   _____ Soft tissue

   Radial/ulnar deviation

   _____ Bony   _____ Capsular   _____ Soft tissue

■ ■ ■ Lab Activities

Student's Name _____ Date Due _____

1. Perform the motions of the elbow and forearm joints with your partner.

    A. Perform a motion and then your partner names the motions you performed.

    B. Your partner names a motion and then you perform that motion.

2. Using the worksheets question 6 for reference, for each of the motions available at the following joints:

    A. Place your open left hand in the correct orientation to represent the plane of a motion.

    B. Place your right index finger to indicate the axis of that motion.

    C. Enter the plane and axis for each motion in the following chart.

Radiocarpal Joint	Plane	Axis
Flexion/extension		
Radial/ulnar deviation		
Circumduction		

3. Observe the amount of motion available at the radiocarpal joint in each plane.

    For each of the motions available at the radioulnar joint, estimate the degrees of motion available by checking the box that *most closely* describes that amount of motion. (Do not measure with a goniometer.)

Motions	0°–45°	46°–90°	91°–135°	136°–180°
Flexion				
Extension				
Radial deviation				
Ulnar deviation				

4. Move your partner's wrist passively through the available range of motion making note of the end feel. If possible repeat with several people. Review question 9 in the worksheets for normal end feel.

    A. Is your partner's end feel consistent with normal end feel for the following:

    _____ Flexion/extension   _____ Radial/ulnar deviation

    B. What structures create the end feel for the following:

    Flexion/extension: _____

    Radial/ulnar deviation: _____

5. On the skeleton, anatomical models, and at least one partner, locate, palpate, and observe the following structures. The reference position is the anatomical position. Having pictures for reference is helpful when trying to find structures. Not all structures can be palpated on your partner.

Radius

Styloid process	Projection at the distal end of the radius. Palpate at the distal lateral aspect of the radius. Note that the radial styloid process lies more distal than the ulnar styloid process. 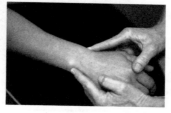 **FIGURE 11-8.** Examiner's right index finger is palpating the radial styloid process.

Ulna

Styloid process	Projection at the distal end of the ulna. Palpate the distal posterior aspect of the ulna. Note that the ulnar styloid process is more prominent than the radial styloid process. See Figure 11-8. Examiner: left index finger is palpating the ulnar styloid process.

Proximal Row of Carpal Bones

Scaphoid	Located in the proximal row of carpal bones. Palpate on the radial side of the wrist just distal to the radial styloid process and in line with the thumb. **FIGURE 11-9.** Palpating the scaphoid.
Lunate	Located in the proximal row of carpal bones in line with the middle finger. Palpate on the dorsal surface by sliding your thumb toward the wrist along the middle metacarpal past the capitate. **FIGURE 11-10.** Palpating the lunate.
Triquetrum	Located in the proximal row of carpal bones on the ulnar side of the wrist just distal to the ulna and in line with the fourth and fifth fingers. The articular disk lies between the ulna and the triquetrum. From palpating the lunate move laterally.

(Continued...)

Proximal Row of Carpal Bones *(continued)*

Pisiform	A small bone that appears to lie on the triquetrum on the anterior surface of the wrist inline with the fifth finger. Palpate it on the palmar surface on the ulnar side. The pisiform is more superficial than the hook of the hamate and is often confused with the hook of the hamate. 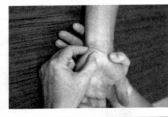 **FIGURE 11-11.** Palpating the pisiform.

Distal Row of Carpal Bones

Trapezium	Located in the distal row of carpal bones on the radial side. It articulates with the first metacarpal bone (thumb). Palpate by moving your thumb proximally along the first metacarpal.
Trapezoid	A small bone just medial to the trapezium in the distal row of carpal bones. It articulates with the second metacarpal bone. Palpate on the dorsal surface by sliding your thumb toward the wrist along the second metacarpal.
Capitate	The largest carpal bone of the distal row. It articulates with the third metacarpal and part of the fourth metacarpal bones. With the wrist in palmar flexion palpate the capitate by moving you thumb proximally along the dorsal surface of the metacarpal bone of the middle finger to an indentation just proximal to the third metacarpal. The capitate lies in this indentation. The capitate can be used as the reference point to locate many of the other carpal bones. **FIGURE 11-12.** Palpating the capitate.
Hamate	Located on the ulnar side of the wrist medial to the capitate and in line with the fourth and fifth metacarpals. Palpate the hamate by grasping it between your thumb and first finger on the ulnar side of the wrist.
Hook of the hamate	The projection on the palmar surface of the hamate. The hook can be palpated using the tip of your thumb with deep pressure applied just medial to the longitudinal arches at the wrist. **FIGURE 11-13.** Palpating the hook of the hamate.

(Continued...)

Other Structures

Radial collateral ligament	Located on the radial side of the wrist. Attachments are the radial styloid process proximally and the scaphoid and trapezium distally. Palpate by placing the pad of one finger over the lateral aspect of the wrist, move the wrist into ulnar deviation, and feel the ligament become taut.
Ulnar collateral ligament	Located on the ulnar side of the wrist. Attachments are the ulnar styloid process proximally and the pisiform and triquetrum distally. Palpate by placing the pad of one finger over the medial aspect of the wrist, move the wrist into radial deviation and feel the ligament become taut.
Palmar radiocarpal ligament	Located on the palmar surface of the wrist deep to the wrist and finger tendons. It is a broad, thick band extending from the anterior surface of the distal radius and ulna to the anterior surface of the scaphoid, lunate, and triquetrum. Palpate by placing your finger pads on the lateral aspect of the palmar surface of the wrist and extend the wrist to make the ligament taut. Palpating is difficult because of the many tendons in the area.
Dorsal radiocarpal ligament	Located on the posterior side of the wrist deep to the wrist and finger extensor tendons. The proximal attachment is on the distal radius, and the distal attachment is the scaphoid, lunate, and triquetrum. This ligament is not as thick as the palmar radiocarpal ligament. Wrist flexion makes the dorsal radiocarpal ligament taut. Palpating is difficult because of the many tendons in the area.
Articular disk	Located on the ulnar side of the wrist between the ulna proximally and the triquetrum distally. Palpate on the ulnar side between the ulna and triquetrum.
Palmar fascia	Also known as the palmar aponeurosis, it is a relatively thick, triangular-shaped fascia located superficially at the midline of the palm of the hand. The palmaris longus tendon and the flexor retinaculum blend into this fascia.
Radiocarpal joint	The articulation of the distal radius with the scaphoid and lunate carpal bones. Palpate on the lateral side of the wrist.
Midcarpal joint	The articulation between the proximal and distal rows of carpal bones. Although not a true joint, it is often considered as such. Palpate the individual bones as previously described.

6. Use a disarticulated skeleton or anatomical model of the radiocarpal joint and apply the rules of joint arthrokinematics and the concave-convex rule to perform the following activities.

   A. Underline the correct answer.

      The radius is: Concave   Convex

      The carpals are: Concave   Convex

   B. Move the distal bone (the proximal row of carpal bones) on the radius in flexion/extension and ulnar/radial deviation.

   C. Observe the movement of the proximal row of carpal bones on the radius. Circle the motions that you observed.

      Roll   Spin   Glide

7. Locate the following on the skeleton, anatomical models, and at least one partner:

A. Locate the origin and insertion of the muscle on the skeleton.

B. Stretch a large rubber band taut by placing one end at the origin and the other end at the insertion of a muscle on the skeleton.

C. Perform the motion that the muscle does and observe how the rubber band becomes less taut and shorter, similar to the muscle shortening as it contracts.

D. Perform the opposite motion and observe how the rubber band becomes tauter and longer, similar to the muscle lengthening as it is being stretched.

E. After locating the muscle on the skeleton, locate the muscle on your partner. The position described for locating the muscle on your partner is the manual muscle test position for a fair or better grade of muscle strength. Not all origins, insertions, and muscle bellies can be palpated on your partner.

F. When possible, palpate the origin, insertion, and muscle belly of each muscle by:

1) Placing your fingers on the origin and insertion, and asking your partner to contract the muscle.

2) Moving your fingers from the origin and insertion over the contracting muscle.

3) Asking your partner to relax the muscle and again moving your fingers from the origin to the insertion over the muscle.

4) Note the difference between the contracting and relaxed muscle.

G. In the following tables, the information needed to palpate each muscle is provided. The information includes position of the person, origin and insertion of the muscle, the line of pull of the muscle, the muscle's action, instructions to give to the person to make the muscle contract, and, finally, information on the best location to palpate the muscle.

Sitting Position

FLEXOR CARPI ULNARIS	Located superficially on the anterior ulnar side of the forearm.
	FIGURE 11-14. Palpating the flexor carpi ulnaris.
Position of person:	Sit with the elbow flexed to 90°, the forearm supinated and supported on a table, and the wrist in the neutral position.
Origin:	Medial epicondyle of the humerus.
Insertion:	Pisiform, hamate, and base of the fifth metacarpal.
Line of pull:	Vertical on the anterior medial surface.
Muscle action:	Wrist flexion, ulnar deviation.
Palpate:	The tendon on the anterior ulnar side of the wrist, and the muscle belly on the anterior ulnar side of the forearm approximately 2 to 3 inches below the elbow.
Instructions to person:	Flex your wrist toward the little finger side lifting your hand off the table.

(Continued...)

FLEXOR CARPI RADIALIS	Located superficially on the anterior forearm.
	FIGURE 11-15. Palpating the flexor carpi radialis.
Position of person:	Sit with the elbow flexed to 90°, the forearm supinated and supported on a table, and the wrist in the neutral position.
Origin:	Medial epicondyle of the humerus.
Insertion:	Base of the second and third metacarpal bones.
Line of pull:	Vertical on the anterior lateral surface.
Muscle action:	Wrist flexion, radial deviation.
Palpate:	The tendon on the anterior radial side of the wrist, and the muscle belly on the anterior and slightly medial surface of the forearm just proximal to the midpoint between the medial epicondyle and the carpometacarpal joint of the thumb. When an individual has a palmaris longus muscle, the flexor carpi radialis tendon lies lateral to the palmaris longus tendon.
Instructions to person:	Flex your wrist toward the thumb side lifting your hand off the table.
PALMARIS LONGUS	Located superficially in the midline of the anterior forearm.
	FIGURE 11-16. Palpating the palmaris longus.
Position of person:	Sit with the elbow flexed to 90°, the forearm supinated and supported on a table, and the wrist in the neutral position.
Origin:	Medial epicondyle of the humerus.
Insertion:	Palmar fascia.
Line of pull:	Vertical on the anterior surface.
Muscle action:	Assists in wrist flexion.
Palpate:	The tendon is in the midline on the anterior surface of the wrist medial to the flexor carpi radialis tendon. This muscle is absent in some individuals bilaterally and some individuals have only one.
Instructions to person:	Flex your wrist lifting your hand off the table.

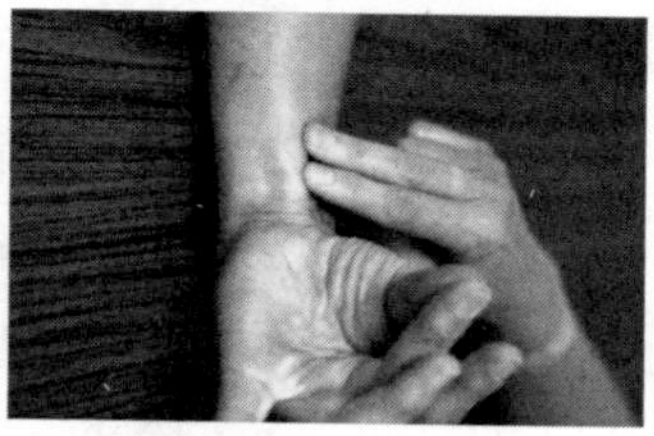

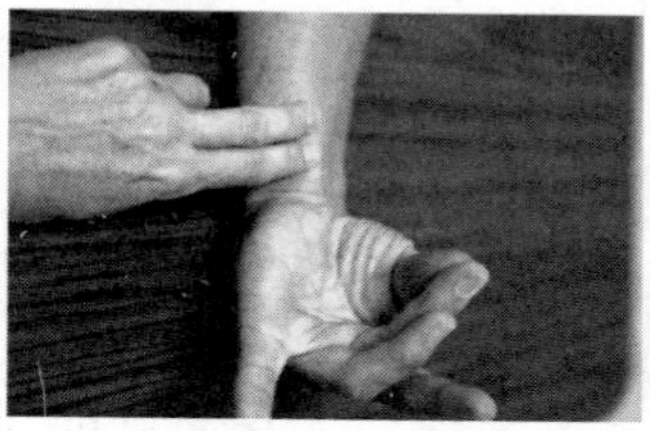

(Continued...)

Sitting Position *(continued)*

EXTENSOR CARPI RADIALIS LONGUS	Located superficially on the posterior radial side of the forearm. **FIGURE 11-17.** Palpating the extensor carpi radialis longus.
Position of person:	Sit with the elbow flexed to 90°, the forearm pronated and supported on a table, and the wrist in the neutral position.
Origin:	Supracondylar ridge of the humerus.
Insertion:	Base of the second metacarpal bone.
Line of pull:	Vertical on the posterior surface.
Muscle action:	Wrist extension, radial deviation.
Palpate:	The tendon on the dorsal side of the wrist proximal to the insertion on the second metacarpal, and the muscle belly on the lateral aspect of the forearm just distal to the elbow.
Instructions to person:	Extend your wrist toward the thumb side by lifting your hand off the table.
EXTENSOR CARPI RADIALIS BREVIS	Located superficially on the posterior radial side of the forearm.
Position of person:	Sit with the elbow flexed to 90°, the forearm pronated and supported on a table, and the wrist in the neutral position.
Origin:	Lateral epicondyle of the humerus.
Insertion:	Base of the third metacarpal bone.
Line of pull:	Vertical on the posterior surface near the midline.
Muscle action:	Wrist extension.
Palpate:	The tendon on the dorsal side of the wrist proximal to the insertion on the metacarpal, and the muscle belly on the lateral aspect posterior side of the proximal forearm.
Instructions to person:	Extend your wrist by lifting your hand off the table.

(Continued...)

EXTENSOR CARPI ULNARIS	Located superficially on the posterior radial side of the forearm.
	 FIGURE 11-18. Palpating the extensor carpi ulnaris.
Position of person:	Sit with the elbow flexed to 90°, the forearm pronated and supported on a table, and the wrist in the neutral position.
Origin:	Lateral epicondyle of the humerus.
Insertion:	Base of the fifth metacarpal.
Line of pull:	Diagonally with a large vertical component on the posterior medial surface.
Muscle action:	Wrist extension, ulnar deviation.
Palpate:	Palpate the tendon on the dorsal ulnar side of the wrist just above the ulnar styloid process, and between the ulnar styloid process and the fifth metacarpal. Palpate the muscle belly on the lateral aspect posterior side of the proximal forearm.
Instructions to person:	Extend your wrist toward the little finger side by lifting your hand off the table.

8. A. Using your <u>right hand</u>, open a jar with a screw-on lid. Does your hand move into radial or ulnar deviation as you loosen the lid? _____

   B. Replace the lid on the jar using your <u>right hand</u>. Does your hand move into radial or ulnar deviation as you tighten the lid? _____

   C. Using your <u>left hand</u>, open a jar with a screw-on lid. Does your hand move into radial or ulnar deviation as you loosen the lid? _____

   D. Replace the lid on the jar using your <u>left hand</u>. Does your hand move into radial or ulnar deviation as you tighten the lid? _____

9. Diagram the lever that describes the activity at the wrist as a mug is lowered to the table when the forearm is supported in midposition on the table.

   A. Draw a stick figure lowering a mug to the table. The person is sitting with the forearm in midposition (between pronation and supination). The wrist is in radial deviation and in neutral (between flexion and extension). The midpoint of the forearm is resting on the edge of the table.

   B. Draw arrows to indicate the direction of the movement, the line of pull of the muscle, and of gravity.

C. Label the arrow that represents force with an "F" and the arrow that represents resistance with an "R."

10. Analyze the activity at the wrist when lowering a mug to the table in the midposition as diagrammed in question 9 by answering the following questions:

   A. The starting range of motion is _____ ° of radial deviation, and the ending

   range of motion is _____ ° of ulna deviation.

   B. What is the "axis" of the motion? _____

   C. Is the movement with or against gravity? _____

   D. Is gravity or muscle the "force" producing the movement? _____

   E. Is gravity or muscle the "resistance" to the movement? _____

   F. Which muscles are the agonists? _____

   G. Which muscles are the antagonists? _____

   H. Is the agonist acting to overcome gravity or to slow down gravity? _____

   I. Is the agonist performing a concentric or an eccentric contraction? _____

   J. Is the antagonist contracting? _____

   K. Is this an open or closed kinetic chain activity? _____

■ ■ ■ Post-Lab Questions

Student's Name _____ Date Due _____

After you have completed the Worksheets and Lab Activities, answer the following questions without using your book or notes. When finished, check your answers.

1. The wrist flexors share a common proximal attachment on, or in the area of, the

   _____ .

2. List the muscles of the wrist that attach on the posterior side of the wrist.

   _____

3. List the two muscles that attach on the base of the fifth metacarpal.

_____

4. Which muscle does not have two bony attachments and what is its nonbony attachment?

_____

5. List the muscles that act together to produce ulnar deviation of the wrist.

_____

6. When the muscles listed on the following table perform the movement listed, list the movement that must be neutralized and list the neutralizing muscles.

Movement and Muscle	Movement to be Neutralized	Neutralizing Muscles
Wrist extension by extensor carpi radialis longus		
Wrist flexion by flexor carpi ulnaris		

7. Can the position of the elbow joint affect the range of motion of the wrist?

_____

Explain your answer. _____

8. Explain why the extensor carpi radialis brevis does not play a major role in wrist radial deviation?

_____

9. An individual with a diagnosis of ulnar nerve entrapment has signs of muscle weakness. Which wrist muscle(s) would be involved?

_____

10. Loss of radial nerve function results in a condition known as "wrist drop." Explain why?

_____

_____

11. Starting on the anterior medial side and proceeding laterally around the wrist, name the wrist muscles in the order encountered.

_____

_____

12. Generally the wrist flexors and extensors are innervated by which nerves?

 A. Wrist extensors: _____

 B. Wrist flexors: _____

 C. List the exception(s): _____

13. In the photograph here (Fig. 11-19) which of the person's wrists does not have a palmaris longus muscle tendon?

 _____Right   _____Left

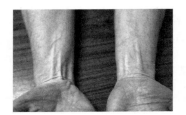

FIGURE 11-19. Palmaris longus.

Hand

■ ■ ■ Worksheets

Student's Name _____ Date Due _____

Complete the following questions prior to the lab class.

1. A. What is the distinction between intrinsic and extrinsic muscles?

   _____

   _____

   B. What is another word for prehension? _____

   C. List the types of prehension.

   _____

   _____

2. On Figures 12-1 through 12-4:

   A. Label the joints and bones:

   Carpometacarpal joints (CMC)   Metacarpophalangeal joints (MCP)
   Interphalangeal joints (DIP, PIP, IP) Metacarpals 1–5
   Phalanges: proximal, middle, distal   Scaphoid
   Lunate   Pisiform
   Hamate   Trapezium
   Trapezoid   Capitate

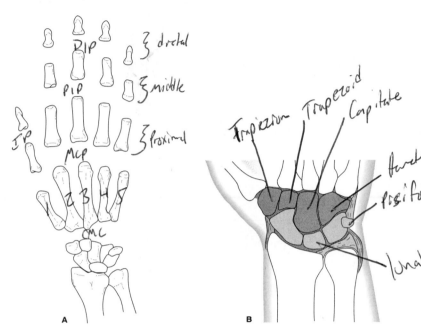

FIGURE 12-1. *(A)* Joints and bones of the hand and wrist. *(B)* Bones of the wrist.

   B. Label the following structures:
   Flexor retinaculum   Palmar carpal ligament
   Transverse carpal ligament

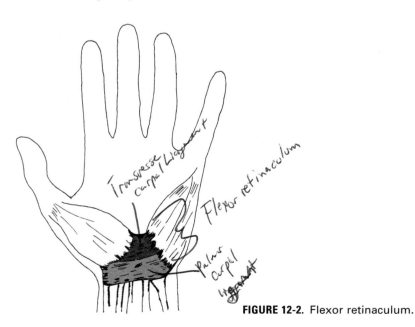

FIGURE 12-2. Flexor retinaculum.

C. Draw in the extensor retinaculum.

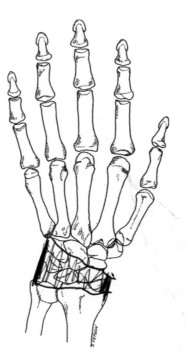

FIGURE 12-3. Extensor retinaculum.

D. Label the following arches:
   Proximal carpal arch
   Longitudinal arch

   Distal carpal arch

longitudinal arch

Proximal carpal arch

Distal Carpal arch

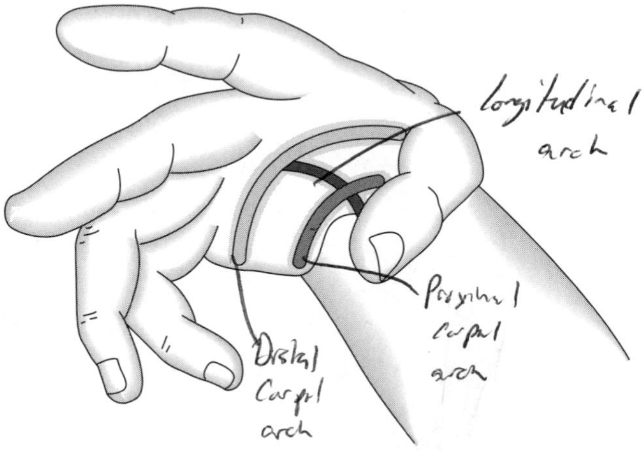

FIGURE 12-4. Arches of hand.

3. On Figures 12-5 through 12-11:
   A. Label the origin and insertion of the muscles listed.
      Color the origin in red and the insertion in blue.
   B. Join the origin and insertion to show the line of pull.

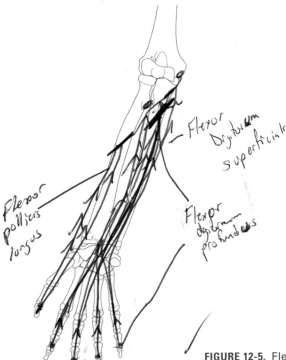

FIGURE 12-5. Flexor digitorum superficialis, flexor digitorum profundus, and flexor pollicis longus.

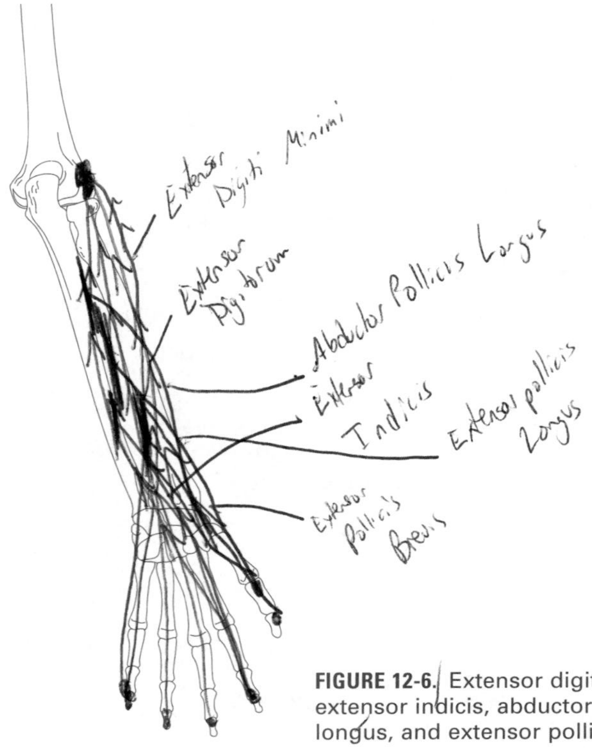

FIGURE 12-6. Extensor digitorum, extensor digiti minimi, extensor indicis, abductor pollicis longus, extensor pollicis longus, and extensor pollicis brevis.

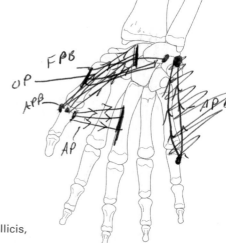

FIGURE 12-7. Flexor pollicis brevis, opponens pollicis, abductor pollicis brevis, and adductor pollicis.

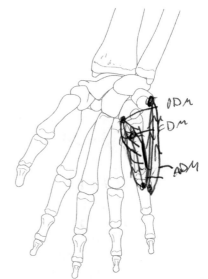

FIGURE 12-8. Opponens digiti minimi, flexor digiti minimi, and abductor digiti minimi.

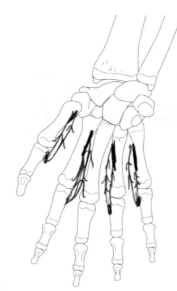

FIGURE 12-9. Palmar interossei.

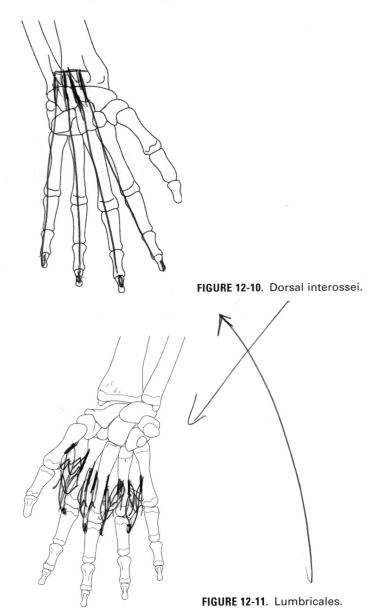

FIGURE 12-10. Dorsal interossei.

FIGURE 12-11. Lumbricales.

4. For each joint listed, identify the following:

Joint	Shape	Degrees of Freedom	Motions	Plane	Axis
Thumb CMC					
Thumb MP					
Thumb IP					
Finger MP					
Finger PIP					
Finger DIP					

5. At each of the following joints, identify which surface is concave and which is convex.

Joint	Concave	Convex
Finger DIP and PIP		
Metacarpophalangeal		
Thumb CMC		
Thumb IP		

6. For each of the joints below provide the close-packed position and the loose-packed position. (Refer to Chapter 4.)

Joint	Close-Packed	Loose-Packed
Finger DIP and PIP		
Metacarpophalangeal		

7. For each of the following joints, describe the end feel. (Refer to Chapter 4 for descriptions.)

Joint	End Feel
Finger DIP and PIP	
Metacarpophalangeal	

8. Match the following ligament and structure with the appropriate function or characteristic. Each term may be used more than once. Each function or characteristic may have more than one answer.

_____ Is located on the anterior surface

_____ Composed of two parts

_____ Is part of the carpal tunnel

_____ Holds tendons close to wrist

_____ Is located on the posterior surface

_____ Is located on the posterior and sides of the proximal phalanges

_____ Provides attachment of extensor tendons to middle and distal phalanges

A. Flexor retinaculum

B. Extensor retinaculum

C. Extensor expansion

D. Transverse carpal ligament

E. Palmar carpal ligament

9. For each muscle listed, check the motions for which the muscle is considered a prime mover for motions of the thumb or fingers.

Muscle	Flexion	Extension	Abduction	Adduction	Opposition
Flexor digitorum superficialis					
Flexor digitorum profundus					
Extensor digitorum					
Extensor digiti minimi					
Extensor indicis					
Abductor pollicis longus					
Extensor pollicis longus					
Extensor pollicis brevis					
Flexor pollicis longus					
Flexor pollicis brevis					
Abductor pollicis brevis					
Opponens pollicis					
Adductor pollicis					
Flexor digiti minimi					
Abductor digiti minimi					
Opponens digiti minimi					
Dorsal interossei					
Palmar interossei					
Lumbricales					

10. Of the extrinsic muscles of the hand:

A. List those that are multijoint muscles.

B. Identify which joints the muscle crosses by placing in the cell the position that lengthens the muscle over that joint.

Muscle	Elbow	Wrist	CMC	MP	PIP	DIP	Thumb IP

11. The tendons of which muscles pass through the carpal tunnel?

_____

_____

12. Which nerve passes through the carpal tunnel?

_____

■ ■ ■ Lab Activities

Student's Name _____ Date Due _____

1. Perform the motions of the thumb and finger joints with your partner.

A. Perform a motion and then your partner names the motion you performed.

B. Your partner names a motion and then you perform that motion.

2. Using the worksheets question 4 for reference, for each of the motions available at the thumb CMC and finger MP joints:

A. Place your open left hand in the correct orientation to represent the plane of a motion.

B. Place your right index finger to indicate the axis of that motion.

3. Observe the amount of motion available at each joint in each plane.

   For each of the motions available at the joints listed, estimate the degrees of motion available by checking the box that *most closely* describes that amount of motion. (Do not measure with a goniometer.)

Thumb Carpometacarpal

Motions	0°–45°	46°–90°	91°–135°	136°–180°
Flexion				
Extension				
Abduction				
Adduction				
Opposition				

Thumb Metacarpalphalangeal

Motions	0°–45°	46°–90°	91°–135°	136°–180°
Flexion				
Extension				

Finger Metacarpalphalangeal

Motions	0°–45°	46°–90°	91°–135°	136°–180°
Flexion				
Extension				
Abduction				
Adduction				

Finger Interphalangeal

Motions	0°–45°	46°–90°	91°–135°	136°–180°
PIP Flexion				
DIP Flexion				

4. Passively move your partner through the available range of motion of the finger IP and MP joints making note of the end feel. If possible repeat with several people. Review question 7 in the worksheets for the normal end feel.

   A. Is your partner's end feel consistent with normal end feel?

B. What structures create the normal end feel for the finger?

MP joint

_____

IP joint

_____

5. Referring to question 10 in the worksheets, assume the positions that lengthen the extrinsic hand muscle simultaneously over the joints they cross.

6. On the skeleton, anatomical models, and at least one partner, locate, palpate, and observe the following structures. The reference position is the anatomical position. Having pictures for reference is helpful when trying to find structures. Not all structures are palpable on your partner.

Thumb

First metacarpal	Palpate by grasping the thumb just above the carpometacarpal joint. Articulates with the trapezium bone and proximal phalange. **FIGURE 12-12.** Palpating first metacarpal.
Proximal phalange	Palpate by grasping the thumb just above the metacarpophalangeal joint. Articulates with the first metacarpal bone and the distal phalange.
Distal phalange	Palpate by grasping the end of the thumb. Articulates with the proximal phalange.
Carpometacarpal joint (CMC)	Palpate the CMC joint on the palmar radial side of the hand at the wrist. The trapezium articulates with the base of the metacarpal. **FIGURE 12-13.** Palpating thumb CMC.
Metacarpophalangeal joint (MP)	Palpate the MP joint at the distal end of the metacarpal as it articulates with the proximal phalange.
Interphalangeal joint (IP)	Palpate the IP joint at the junction of the proximal and distal phalanges.

Fingers: Digits 2–5

Metacarpals	Palpate on the dorsum of the hand. The long bones of the hand that lie between the wrist and the fingers. The bases of the metacarpals articulate with the distal row of the carpal bones. The heads of the metacarpals articulate with the proximal phalanges of the fingers. **FIGURE 12-14.** Palpating the metacarpals.
Proximal phalange	Palpate by grasping a finger just distal to the MP joints of the fingers.
Middle phalange	Palpate by grasping a finger between the IP joints.
Distal phalange	Palpate by grasping the end of a finger distal to the DIP joint.
Carpometacarpal joint (CMC)	Palpate on the dorsum of the hand by moving proximally on the metacarpals. This is the articulation of the distal row of carpal bones with the metacarpals. **FIGURE 12-15.** Palpating the CMC.
Metacarpophalangeal joint (MP)	Also called "knuckles," these joints are palpated by grasping the metacarpal with one hand and the adjunct proximal phalange with the other hand. Move the phalange on the metacarpal noting where the motion occurs. Move the hand from the metacarpal to the area in which the motion is occurring.
Proximal interphalangeal joint (PIP)	Palpate by stabilizing the proximal phalange with one hand and grasping the middle phalange with the other hand. Move the middle phalange on the proximal phalange noting where the motion occurs. Move the hand from the proximal phalange to the area in which the motion is occurring.
Distal interphalangeal joint (DIP)	Palpate by stabilizing the middle phalange with one hand and grasping the distal phalange with the other hand moving the distal phalange on the middle phalange noting were the motion occurs. Move the hand from the middle phalange to the area in which the motion is occurring.

7. Use a disarticulated skeleton or anatomical model of the following joints and apply the rules of joint arthrokinematics and the concave-convex rule to perform the following activities.

Thumb Carpometacarpal Joint

A. Underline the correct answer.

   The trapezium is: Concave   Convex

   The metacarpal is: Concave   Convex

B. Move the metacarpal on the trapezium in all planes of motion permitted by the joint.

C. When the metacarpal moves on the trapezium what arthrokinematic motions occur.

Roll   Spin   Glide

Thumb and Finger Metacarpophalangeal Joints

A. Underline the correct answer.

The metacarpal is: Concave   Convex

The phalange is: Concave   Convex

B. Move the phalange on the metacarpal in all planes of motion permitted by the joint.

C. When the proximal phalange moves on the metacarpal what arthrokinematic motions occur.

Roll   Spin   Glide

Finger Interphalangeal Joints

A. Underline the correct answer.

The proximal phalange is: Concave   Convex

The middle phalange is: Concave   Convex

B. Move the middle phalange on the proximal phalange in all planes of motion permitted by the joint.

C. When the middle phalange moves on the proximal phalange what arthrokinematic motions occur.

Roll   Spin   Glide

8. Locate the following on the skeleton, anatomical models, and at least one partner:

A. Locate the origin and insertion of the muscle on the skeleton.

B. Stretch a large rubber band taut by placing one end at the origin and the other end at the insertion of a muscle on the skeleton.

C. Perform the motion that the muscle does and observe how the rubber band becomes less taut and shorter, similar to the muscle shortening as it contracts.

D. Perform the opposite motion and observe how the rubber band becomes more taut and longer, similar to the muscle lengthening as it is being stretched.

E. After locating the muscle on the skeleton, locate the muscle on your partner. The position described for locating the muscle on your partner is the manual muscle test position for a fair or better grade of muscle strength. Not all origins, insertions, and muscle bellies can be palpated on your partner.

F. When possible, palpate the origin, insertion, and muscle belly of each muscle by:

1) Placing your fingers on the origin and insertion, and asking your partner to contract the muscle.

2) Moving your fingers from the origin and insertion over the contracting muscle.

3) Asking your partner to relax the muscle and again moving your fingers from the origin to the insertion over the muscle.

4) Note the difference between the contracting and relaxed muscle.

G. In the following tables, the information needed to palpate each muscle is provided. The information includes position of the person, origin and insertion of the muscle, the line of pull of the muscle, the muscle's action, instructions to give to the person to make the muscle contract, and, finally, information on the best location to palpate the muscle.

Sitting Position with the Elbow Flexed to 90° and the Forearm Supported on a Table

FLEXOR DIGITORUM SUPERFICIALIS	On the anterior surface, located deep to the wrist flexors and the palmaris longus.
Position of person:	Forearm supinated, and wrist and fingers in neutral.
Origin:	Common flexor tendon on the medial epicondyle of the humerus, coranoid process, and radius.
Insertion:	Each side of the middle phalange of the four fingers.
Line of pull:	Vertical on the anterior surface.
Muscle action:	Flexes the MCP and PIP joints of the fingers.
Palpate:	The tendon at the wrist lateral and deep to the palmaris longus, and the muscle belly on the anterior surface of the forearm distal to the elbow.
Instructions to person:	Bend the first two joints of your fingers so that the pads of the fingers rests against your palm.
FLEXOR DIGITORUM PROFUNDUS	Located deep to the flexor digitorum superficialis on the anterior surface of the forearm and hand.
Position of person:	Forearm supinated, and wrist and fingers in neutral.
Origin:	Upper three-quarters of the ulna.
Insertion:	Distal phalange of the four fingers.
Line of pull:	Mostly vertical on the anterior surface.
Muscle action:	Flexes MCP, PIP, and DIP joints of the fingers.
Palpate:	Difficult to palpate the tendon as it is deep to other tendons, and the muscle belly is on the anterior surface of the forearm distal to the elbow.
Instructions to person:	Curl your fingers into your palm.
EXTENSOR DIGITORUM	Located superficially on the posterior forearm and hand.

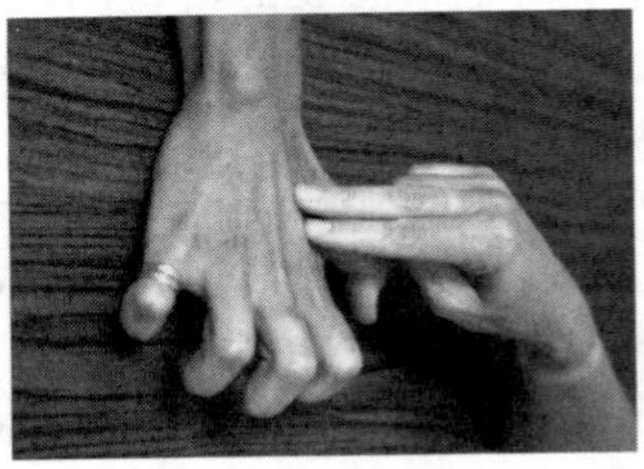

FIGURE 12-16. Palpating the extensor digitorum tendons.

Position of person:	Forearm pronated, and wrist and fingers in neutral.
Origin:	Lateral epicondyle of the humerus.
Insertion:	Base of the distal phalange of fingers 2–5.

(Continued...)

Line of pull:	Mostly vertical on the posterior surface.
Muscle action:	Extends the MCP, PIP, and DIP joints of the fingers.
Palpate:	The tendons can be palpated on the dorsum of the hand, and the muscle bellies are palpated on the proximal posterior lateral forearm.
Instructions to person:	Straighten and lift your fingers off the table.
EXTENSOR DIGITI MINIMI	Located deep to the extensor digitorum and extensor carpi ulnaris muscles at its origin. Located superficially on the posterior medial surface of the wrist.
Position of person:	Forearm pronated, and wrist and fifth finger in neutral.
Origin:	Lateral epicondyle of the humerus.
Insertion:	Base of the distal phalange of the fifth finger.
Line of pull:	Mostly vertical on the posterior surface.
Muscle action:	Extends the MCP, PIP, and DIP joints of the fifth finger.
Palpate:	On the dorsum of the hand over the fifth metacarpal lateral to the extensor digitorum.
Instructions to person:	Straighten and lift your little finger.
EXTENSOR INDICIS	Located deep on the posterior lateral surface of the forearm.
Position of person:	Forearm pronated and wrist and index finger in neutral.
Origin:	Posterior surface of distal ulna.
Insertion:	The base of the distal phalange via the extensor hood.
Line of pull:	Mostly vertical on the posterior surface.
Muscle action:	Extends the MCP, PIP, and DIP joints of the index finger.
Palpate:	The tendon on the dorsum of the hand over the second metacarpal medial to the tendon of the extensor digitorum, and the muscle belly on the posterior distal ulna.
Instructions to person:	Straighten and lift your index finger off the table.
FLEXOR POLLICIS LONGUS	Located deep on the anterior surface of the forearm.
Position of person:	Forearm supinated, and the wrist in neutral, the thumb resting on the palm over the second metacarpal.
Origin:	Anterior surface of the radius.

(Continued...)

Sitting Position *(continued)*

Insertion:	Distal phalange of the thumb.
Line of pull:	Mostly vertical.
Muscle action:	Flexes the CMC, MCP, and IP joints of the thumb.
Palpate:	The tendon on the palmar surface of the proximal phalange, and the muscle belly on the anterior surface of the radius about two-thirds of distance from the elbow.
Instructions to person:	Curl your thumb into your palm.
ABDUCTOR POLLICIS LONGUS	Located deep on the posterior forearm. **FIGURE 12-17.** Palpating the abductor pollicis longus.
Position of person:	Forearm supinated, wrist in neutral, thumb resting against the palm over the second metacarpal.
Origin:	Posterior surface of the radius, interosseous membrane, and posterior lateral surface of the middle portion of the ulna.
Insertion:	Radial side of the base of the first metacarpal.
Line of pull:	Mostly vertical.
Muscle action:	Abducts the thumb.
Palpate:	The tendon at the insertion. This tendon lies next to the extensor pollicis brevis tendon to make up the lateral border of the anatomical snuffbox.
Instructions to person:	Lift your thumb off your palm.
EXTENSOR POLLICIS LONGUS	Located deep on the posterior forearm.
Position of person:	Forearm in midposition, wrist and thumb in neutral.
Origin:	Posterior lateral side of the ulna and the interosseous membrane.
Insertion:	Base of the distal phalange of the thumb.
Line of pull:	Vertical.
Muscle action:	Extends the CMC, MCP, and IP joints of the thumb.
Palpate:	The tendon on the dorsum of the proximal phalange. The extensor pollicis longus tendon is on the index finger side of the anatomical snuffbox.

(Continued...)

Instructions to person:	Move your thumb out to the side.
EXTENSOR POLLICIS BREVIS	Located deep on the posterior distal forearm.
Position of person:	Forearm in midposition and the wrist in neutral.
Origin:	Posterior distal surface of the radius.
Insertion:	Base of the proximal phalange of the thumb.
Line of pull:	Mostly vertical.
Muscle action:	Extends the CMC and MCP joints of the thumb.
Palpate:	The tendon at the insertion. This tendon is on the thumb side of the anatomical snuffbox.
Instructions to person:	Move your thumb out to the side.
FLEXOR POLLICIS BREVIS	Located superficially in the thenar group.
Position of person:	Forearm supinated, and the wrist and thumb in neutral.
Origin:	Trapezium, trapezoid, capitate, and flexor retinaculum.
Insertion:	Base of the proximal phalange of the thumb.
Line of pull:	Vertical.
Muscle action:	Flexes the CMC and MCP joints while maintaining the IP joint extended.
Palpate:	The muscle belly in the middle of the thenar group proximal to the metacarpophalangeal joint.
Instructions to person:	Bend your thumb into your palm keeping the last joint of your thumb straight.
ABDUCTOR POLLICIS BREVIS	Located superficially in the thenar group.
Position of person:	Forearm supinated, the wrist in neutral, and thumb resting on the palmar surface of the second metacarpal.
Origin:	Scaphoid, trapezium, and the flexor retinaculum.
Insertion:	Radial side of the base of the proximal phalanx.
Line of pull:	Vertical.
Muscle action:	Abducts the thumb.
Palpate:	The muscle belly in the thenar group on the lateral side of the first metacarpal.
Instructions to person:	Lift your thumb off your palm.

(Continued...)

Sitting Position *(continued)*

OPPONENS POLLICIS	Located deep in the palm.
Position of person:	Forearm supinated, and the wrist and thumb in neutral.
Origin:	Trapezium and flexor retinaculum.
Insertion:	First metacarpal.
Line of pull:	Diagonal and wrapping around the bone, making it spiral.
Muscle action:	Opposes the thumb and little finger by touching the pad of the thumb to the pad of the little finger. Thumb moves out in abduction and around in flexion = opposition.
Palpate:	On the radial side of the first metacarpal lateral to the abductor pollicis brevis.
Instructions to person:	Touch the pad of your thumb to the pad of your little finger.
ADDUCTOR POLLICIS	Located deep in the palm.
Position of person:	Forearm pronated with the hand off the edge of the table, the wrist in neutral, and the thumb in abduction.
Origin:	Capitate, base of the second metacarpal, and palmar surface of the metacarpal.
Insertion:	Base of the proximal phalange of the thumb.
Line of pull:	Horizontal.
Muscle action:	Adducts the thumb by bringing it toward the palm.
Palpate:	In the web space between the first and second metacarpals.
Instructions to person:	Move your thumb into your palm.
FLEXOR DIGITI MINIMI	Located in the hypothenar group.
Position of person:	Forearm supinated, and the wrist and fifth finger in neutral.
Origin:	Hamate and flexor retinaculum.
Insertion:	Base of the proximal phalange of the fifth finger.
Line of pull:	Vertical.
Muscle action:	Flexes the CMC and MCP joints of the fifth finger.
Palpate:	In the hypothenar eminence on the anterior surface over the distal end of the fifth metacarpal.

(Continued...)

Instructions to person:	Curl your little finger into your palm.
ABDUCTOR DIGITI MINIMI	Located superficially on the ulnar border of the hypothenar eminence.
Position of person:	Forearm supinated, and wrist and fifth finger in neutral.
Origin:	Pisiform and tendon of the flexor carpi ulnaris.
Insertion:	Medial side of the base of the proximal phalange of the fifth finger.
Line of pull:	Vertical.
Muscle action:	Abducts the fifth finger.
Palpate:	The muscle belly on the medial aspect of the fifth finger.
Instructions to person:	Move your little finger out to the side.
OPPONENS DIGITI MINIMI	Located deep to the other hypothenar muscles.
Position of person:	Forearm supinated, and the wrist and fifth finger in neutral.
Origin:	Hamate and flexor retinaculum.
Insertion:	Medial side of the fifth metacarpal.
Line of pull:	Diagonal and wrapping around the bone making it spiral.
Muscle action:	Opposes the fifth finger by touching the pad of the fifth finger to the pad of the thumb. Finger moves out in abduction and around in flexion = opposition.
Palpate:	In the hypothenar eminence on the anterior surface over the proximal end of the fifth metacarpal.
Instructions to person:	Touch the pad of your little finger to the pad of your thumb.
DORSAL INTEROSSEI (DI)	Located deep on the dorsum of the hand. 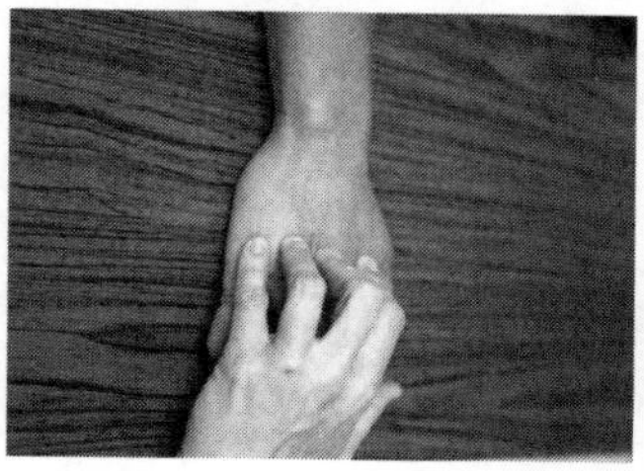 **FIGURE 12-18.** Palpating over the area of the muscle bellies of the dorsal interossei.
Position of person:	Forearm pronated, and the wrist and fingers in neutral.

(Continued...)

Sitting Position *(continued)*

Origin:	1st DI: 1st and 2nd metacarpals. 2nd DI: 2nd and 3rd metacarpals. 3rd DI: 3rd and 4th metacarpals. 4th DI: 4th and 5th metacarpals.
Insertion:	1st DI: Lateral side of proximal phalange of index finger. 2nd DI: Lateral side of proximal phalange of middle finger. 3rd DI: Medial side of proximal phalange of middle finger. 4th DI: Medial side of proximal phalange of ring finger.
Line of pull:	Vertical.
Muscle action:	1st DI: Abducts index finger. 2nd DI: Abducts middle finger laterally. 3rd DI: Abducts middle finger medially. 4th DI: Abducts ring finger.
Palpate:	1st DI: At the base of the proximal phalange of the index finger; the remaining dorsal interossei cannot be palpated.
Instructions to person:	Spread your fingers apart.
PALMAR INTEROSSEI (PI)	Located deep in the palm.
Position of person:	Forearm supinated, and the wrist and fingers in neutral.
Origin:	1st PI: 1st metacarpal. 2nd PI: 2nd metacarpal. 3rd PI: 4th metacarpal. 4th PI: 5th metacarpal.
Insertion:	1st PI: Medial side of proximal phalange of thumb. 2nd PI: Medial side of proximal phalange of index finger. 3rd PI: Lateral side of proximal phalange of ring finger. 4th PI: Lateral side of proximal phalange of fifth finger.
Line of pull:	Vertical.
Muscle action:	1st PI: Adducts thumb. 2nd PI: Adducts the index finger. 3rd PI: Adducts the ring finger. 4th PI: Adducts the fifth finger.
Palpate:	These muscles cannot be palpated.
Instructions to person:	Squeeze your fingers together.
LUMBRICALES	Located deep on the lateral sides of the MP joints.
Position of person:	Forearm supinated, wrist and fingers in neutral.

(Continued...)

Sitting Position *(continued)*

Origin:	Tendons of the flexor digitorum profundus muscle.
Insertion:	Radial side of the corresponding digit's extensor hood.
Line of pull:	Vertical.
Muscle action:	Flexes the MP joints and simultaneously extends the IP joints.
Palpate:	These small deep muscles cannot be palpated.
Instructions to person:	Starting from a hook grasp position, move your fingers in the opposite directions—bend at the first joint and straighten the other joints.

9. Identify the muscle tendons that make up the anatomical snuff box illustrated in Figure 12-19.

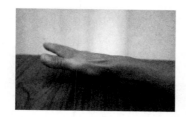

FIGURE 12-19. Anatomical snuff box.

10. Note the amount of wrist motions in each of the following activities:

    A. With fingers flexed, extend the wrist.

    B. With fingers extended, extend the wrist.

    Which position of the fingers permitted more wrist extension? _____

    Why? _____

    C. With the fingers extended, flex the wrist.

    D. With the fingers flexed, flex the wrist.

    Which position of the fingers permitted more wrist flexion? _____

    Why? _____

    How can you determine if active or passive insufficiency limits the range of motion?

    _____

    _____

11. Perform each of the following types of grasp. Describe one functional task performed with each type of grasp. Do not use the examples in the book.

Power Grips

Grip	Description	Example
Cylindrical	All the fingers flex around an object that usually lies at right angle to the forearm.	
Spherical	All the fingers and thumb are abducted and then flexed around an object.	
Hook	The IP joints of the fingers are flexed and the thumb does not participate.	

Precision Grips

Grip	Description	Example
Pad-to-pad	Pad of thumb is touched to pad of a finger; MCP and PIP joints of the fingers are flexed; thumb is adducted and the distal IP joints of both are extended.	
Pinch	A pad-to-pad grip involving the thumb and usually the index finger.	
Three jaw chuck	Pad-to-pad grip involving the thumb, and index and middle fingers.	
Tip-to-tip or Pincer	Tip of the thumb is touched against the tip of another digit.	
Pad-to-side or Lateral prehension	Pad of the extended thumb presses an object against the radial side of the index finger.	
Side-to-side	Two adjacent fingers are adducted.	
Lumbrical or plate	MCP joints flex and the PIP and DIP joints extend; thumb opposes the fingers.	

12. Describe the conditions that permit the extensor muscles of the wrist to produce grasp.

   _____

   _____

   This tendon action of a muscle is also known as: _____

13. Hold a piece of paper between your index and middle fingers (or any two adjacent fingers) while your classmate tries to pull the paper out from between your fingers.

   A. Could the paper be removed easily?

   _____

   B. Which muscles were at work and what were their actions? _____

   _____

   C. Damage to which nerve weakens these muscles? _____

■ ■ ■ **Post-Lab Questions**

Student's Name _____ Date Due _____

After you have completed the Worksheets and Lab Activities, answer the following questions without using your book or notes. When finished, check your answers.

1. Identify the following muscles by their location to each other.

   A. What is the most superficial muscle on the anterior surface of the wrist located in the midline of the wrist?

   _____

   B. What muscle or tendon lies directly underneath the muscle identified in A?

   _____

   C. What muscle or tendon lies directly underneath the muscle identified in B?

   _____

2. What is the difference between an extrinsic muscle and an intrinsic muscle?

   _____

3. Are the thenar and hypothenar muscles intrinsic or extrinsic muscles?

   _____

4. A. List the muscles that make up the anatomical snuffbox.

   _____

   B. Are these muscles intrinsic or extrinsic muscles? _____

5. Which muscle attaches to the tendons of the flexor digitorum profundus and extensor digitorum muscles?

   _____

6. A. Thenar muscles control what structure? _____

   B. The muscles of the thenar muscle group are: _____

   _____

   C. Which nerve innervates the thenar muscle group? _____

   D. Which thumb motions would be affected by damage to this nerve? _____

7. If one were to generalize about the innervation of the muscles of the hand by their location, the muscles on the:

   A. Posterior surface are innervated by the _____

   B. Anterior medial surface are innervated by the _____

   C. Anterior lateral surface are innervated by the _____

8. Injury to which nerve eliminates thumb opposition?

9. Which muscles have the combined action of MP and IP extension?

10. What is the reference point for MP abduction and adduction of the fingers?

11. A. Compared to the fingers, what bone is the thumb missing?

    B. What is the effect of this missing bone on the number of joints?

    C. What motion does the thumb have that fingers 2–4 do not have?

12. All joints of the thumb and fingers are what types of joints?

13. A. Which extrinsic muscles are involved in finger extension? _____

    B. Which extrinsic muscles are involved in finger flexion? _____

14. Name the muscle that abducts the index finger. _____

Clinical Kinesiology and Anatomy of the Trunk

Chapter 13

Temporomandibular Joint

Worksheets

Student's Name ______________________ Date Due ______________

Complete the following questions prior to the lab class.

1. Define the following terms:

   Protrusion: ______________________

   Retrusion or retraction: ______________________

   Lateral deviation: ______________________

2. On Figures 13-1 through 13-4, label the following bones and landmarks:

MANDIBLE:	Angle	Body	Condyle	Coronoid process
	Neck	Notch	Ramus	

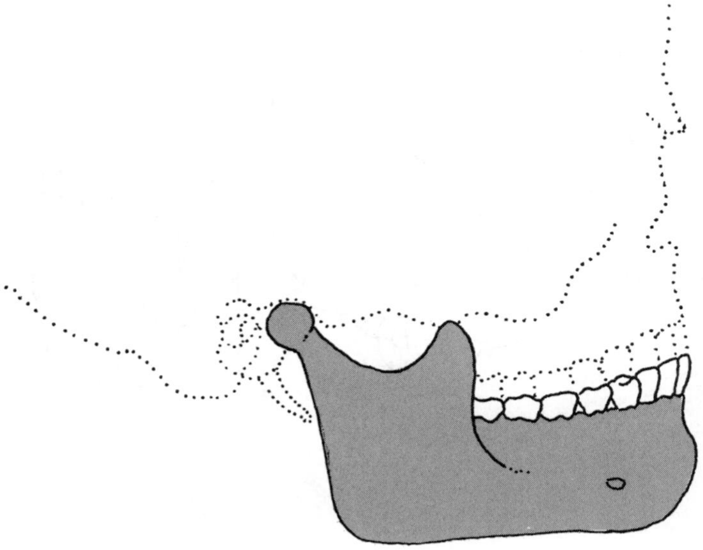

FIGURE 13-1. Mandible, right lateral view.

LANDMARKS: Articular tubercle   Articular fossa   Postglenoid tubercle
                Styloid process   Mastoid process   External auditory meatus
                Zygomatic arch

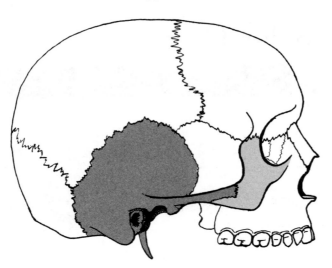

FIGURE 13-2. Landmarks.

SPHENOID: Greater wing of sphenoid   Lateral pterygoid plate of sphenoid
MAXILLA: Maxillary tuberosity

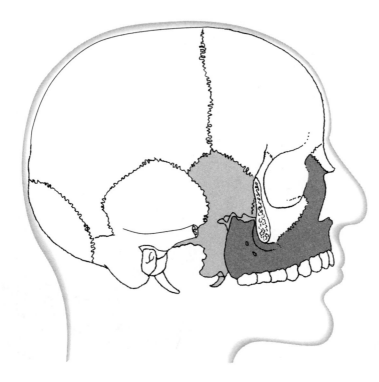

FIGURE 13-3. Lateral view of skull, mandible and zygomatic bones removed.

Temporomandibular joint   Hyoid bone   Thyroid cartilage   Epiglottis
First cricoid ring   Trachea   Stylohyoid ligament   Styloid process

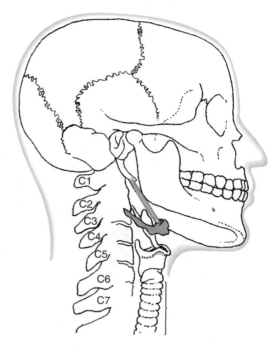

FIGURE 13-4. Lateral view of skull, vertebral column, and trachea.

3. On Figure 13-5, draw in the temporal fossa and label the bones that are part of it.

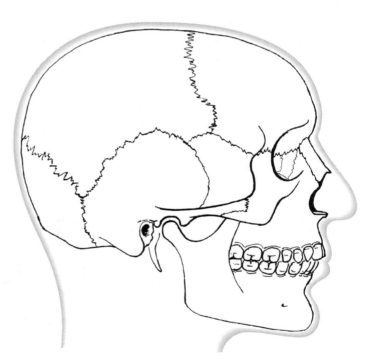

FIGURE 13-5. Temporal fossa.

4. On Figure 13-6, label the following structures:

Lateral ligament (temporomandibular ligament)   Stylomandibular ligament
Sphenomandibular ligament   Joint capsule

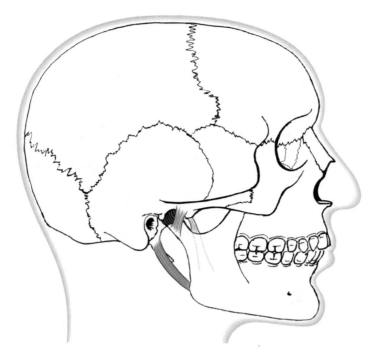

FIGURE 13-6. Lateral view.

5. On Figures 13-7 and 13-8:

   A. Label the origin and insertion of the muscles listed.

   B. Join the origin and insertion to show the line of pull.

   Temporalis   Masseter

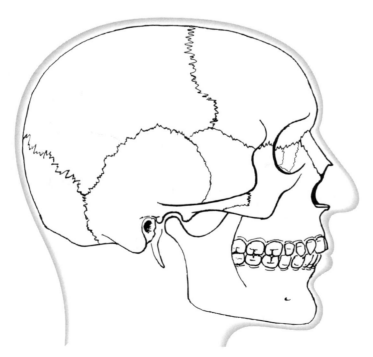

FIGURE 13-7. Lateral view.

C. Identify the medial and lateral pterygoid muscles in Figure 13-8 and label the origin and insertion of each.

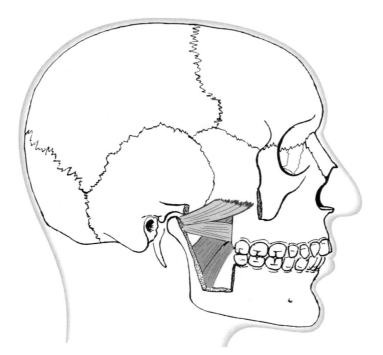

FIGURE 13-8. Medial and lateral pterygoid muscles.

6. For the temporomandibular joint give the following information:

Joint	Shape	Degrees of Freedom	Motions
TMJ			

7. At the temporomandibular joint, identify which surface is concave and which is convex.

Joint	Concave	Convex
TMJ		

8. For the temporomandibular joint provide the close-packed position and the loose-packed position. (Refer to Chapter 4.)

Joint	Close-Packed	Loose-Packed
TMJ		

9. For the temporomandibular joint describe the normal end feel. (Refer to Chapter 4 for descriptions.)

   For elevation (mouth closing):

   _____ Bony   _____ Capsular   _____ Soft tissue approximation

   For all other motions:

   _____ Bony   _____ Capsular   _____ Soft tissue approximation

10. Describe the shape and function of the articular disk of the TMJ.

   _____

   _____

■ ■ ■ Lab Activities

Student's Name _____ Date Due _____

1. Perform the motions of the temporomandibular joint with your partner.
   A. Perform a motion and then your partner names the motions you performed.
   B. Your partner states a motion and then you perform that motion.

2. Observe the amount of motion in each direction at the temporomandibular joint. Motion of the TMJ is often measured with a ruler and recorded in inches or millimeters. For each of the motions available at the TMJ joint, estimate the amount of motion available.

Motions	Inches/Millimeters
Protrusion	
Depression (opening)	
Lateral deviation to one side	

3. Individuals often have difficulty allowing passive movement of the mandible. Passively move your partner through the available range of motion making note of the end feel. If possible repeat with several people. Review question 9 in the preceding section about the normal end feels for the motions of the TMJ.
   A. Is your partner's end feel consistent with normal end feel?

   _____

   B. What structures create the end feel for this joint?

   _____

   _____

4. On the skeleton, anatomical models, and at least one partner, locate, palpate, and observe the structures that follow. The reference position is the anatomical position. Having pictures for reference is helpful when trying to find structures. Not all structures are palpable on your partner.

TMJ	Located just anterior to the middle anterior part of the ear. Palpate the depression between the mandibular condyle and temporal fossa as your partner opens his or her mouth.
	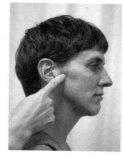
	FIGURE 13-9. Palpating the TMJ.

Mandible or Mandibular Bone

Angle	Located between the body and ramus, it is the joining point of these two landmarks. Palpate by placing one finger on the posterior vertical surface of the mandible below the ear and another finger on the posterior horizontal surface. The point (angle) between your fingers is the angle.
	FIGURE 13-10. Palpating the angle of the mandible.
Body	The horizontal portion of the mandible. The superior surface of the body holds the teeth. Palpate below the lower teeth on the flat jaw line.
	FIGURE 13-11. Palpating the body of the mandible.
Condyle or Condylar process	Posterior projection on the ramus that articulates with the temporal bone. Palpate just anterior to the ear canal and inferior to the zygomatic arch while the mouth is opened and while the mouth is closed.

(Continued...)

Mandible or Mandibular Bone *(continued)*

Coronoid process	Located anterior to the condyle on the ramus. It is the attachment for the masseter muscle. Palpate below the zygomatic arch while the mouth is fully opened. When the mouth is closed, the process moves under the arch and cannot be palpated.
Mental spine	Located on the interior side of the mandible near the midline. It is the attachment for the geniohyoid muscle. Cannot be palpated.
Neck	Located just inferior to the condyle and can be palpated there.
Notch	Located between the condyle and coronoid process on the ramus. Palpate on the ramus of the mandible between the condyle and coronoid process when the mouth is fully open.
Ramus	The vertical portion of the mandible from the angle to the condyle. Palpate on the mandible between the condyle and the angle.

Temporal Bone

Articular tubercle	The anterior portion of the articulating surface of the temporal bone. Difficult to palpate because of overlying muscles.
Articular fossa or Mandibular fossa	Located anterior to the external auditory meatus and articulates with the condyle of the mandible. Palpate when the mouth opens, but it is not easily palpated.
Postglenoid tubercle	The posterior wall of the fossa just anterior to the external auditory meatus. Not easily palpated because of overlying muscles.
Styloid process	A slender projection positioned down and forward from the temporal bone on the inferior, slightly interior surface. It is the attachment for muscles and ligaments. Palpate behind the earlobe between the mastoid process and ramus of mandible; it is difficult to palpate because of overlying muscles.
Mastoid process	Large bony prominence posterior and inferior to the ear. It is an attachment for digastric and sternocleidomastoid muscles. Palpate just posterior to the ear. **FIGURE 13-12.** Palpating the mastoid process.
External auditory meatus	External opening for the ear, located posterior to the TMJ. View from lateral side of head.
Zygomatic process	Posterior portion of the zygomatic arch. It is the attachment for the masseter. Palpate just anterior to the ear on the zygomatic arch.

Sphenoid Bone

Because the sphenoid is located inside the cranium, none of the following structures can be palpated.

Greater wing	Large bony process located medial to the zygomatic bone and arch, and anterior to the rest of the temporal bone. It is the attachment for the temporalis and lateral pterygoid muscles.
Lateral pterygoid plate	Deep to the zygomatic arch. It is the attachment for the lateral and medial pterygoid muscles.
Spine	Deep to the articular fossa of the temporal bone. It is the attachment for the sphenomandibular ligament

Combination of Skull Bones

Temporal fossa	Bony floor formed by zygomatic, frontal, parietal, sphenoid, and temporal bones. It is the attachment of the temporalis muscle. Palpate the general area of the fossa above the ear and zygomatic arch.
Zygomatic arch	Formed by the zygomatic process of the temporal bone posteriorly and the temporal process of the zygomatic bone anteriorly. Palpate anterior to the external auditory meatus between the temporalis and zygomatic bones along the arch. **FIGURE 13-13.** Palpating the zygomatic arch.

Maxilla or Maxillary Bone

Tuberosity	Rounded projection located on the inferior posterior angle. It is the attachment for the medial pterygoid. Cannot be palpated.

Other Structures

Hyoid bone	Horseshoe-shaped bone lying superior to the thyroid cartilage at about the C3 level. It is the attachment for the stylohyoid ligaments, tongue, suprahyoid, and infrahyoid muscles. Palpate on either side of the trachea parallel to the jaw. Notice how it elevates when your partner swallows. **FIGURE 13-14.** Palpating the hyoid bone.

(Continued...)

Other Structures *(continued)*

Thyroid cartilage or "Adam's apple"	Inferior to the hyoid bone at about the C3 to C4 level. It is the attachment for the infrahyoid muscles. This structure is more pronounced in males than females. Palpate in the midline below the hyoid bone.
Lateral ligament or temporomandibular ligament	Attaches on the neck of the mandibular condyle and disk, and then runs superiorly to the articular tubercle of the temporal bone. Cannot be palpated.
Sphenomandibular ligament	Attaches to the spine of the sphenoid bone and runs to the middle of the ramus on the internal surface of the mandible. Cannot be palpated.
Stylomandibular ligament	Attaches to the styloid process of the temporal bone and to the posterior inferior border of the ramus of the mandible. Cannot be palpated.
Stylohyoid ligament	Attaches to the styloid process of the temporal bone and the hyoid bone. Deep to muscles and cannot be palpated.
Joint capsule	Envelops the TMJ. Attaches superiorly to the articular tubercle and borders of the temporal bone, and inferiorly to the neck of the condyle of the mandible. Cannot be palpated.
Articular disk	Attached circumferentially to the capsule and tendon of the lateral pterygoid. Palpate by placing a finger in the external auditory meatus while your partner opens/closes his or her mouth.

5. Use a disarticulated skeleton or anatomical model of the temporomandibular joint and apply the rules of joint arthrokinematics and the concave-convex rule to perform the following activities.

   A. Underline the correct answer.

   The temporal bone is: Concave   Convex

   The mandible condyle is: Concave   Convex

   B. Move the mandible on the temporal bone in all planes of motion.

   C. Observe the movement of the mandible on the temporal bone. Circle the motions that you observe.

   Roll   Spin   Glide

6. Locate the following on the skeleton, anatomical models, and at least one partner:

   A. Locate the origin and insertion of the muscle on the skeleton.

   B. Stretch a large rubber band taut by placing one end at the origin and the other end at the insertion of a muscle on the skeleton.

   C. Perform the motion that the muscle does and observe how the rubber band becomes less taut and shorter, similar to the muscle shortening as it contracts.

   D. Perform the opposite motion and observe how the rubber band becomes more taut and longer, similar to the muscle lengthening as it is being stretched.

   E. After locating the muscle on the skeleton, locate the muscle on your partner. The position described for locating the muscle on your partner is the manual muscle test position for a fair or better grade of muscle strength. Not all origins, insertions, and muscle bellies can be palpated on your partner.

F. When possible, palpate the origin, insertion, and muscle belly of each muscle by:

1) Placing your fingers on the origin and insertion, and asking your partner to contract the muscle.

2) Moving your fingers from the origin and insertion over the contracting muscle.

3) Asking your partner to relax the muscle and again moving your fingers from the origin to the insertion over the muscle.

4) Note the difference between the contracting and relaxed muscle.

G. In the tables that follow, the information needed to palpate each muscle is provided. The information includes position of the person, origin and insertion of the muscle, the line of pull of the muscle, the muscle's action, instructions to give to the person to make the muscle contract, and, finally, information on the best location to palpate the muscle.

Sitting Postion

TEMPORALIS	Superficial on the lateral aspect of the skull.
	 FIGURE 13-15. Palpating the temporalis.
Position of person:	Mouth open.
Origin:	Temporal fossa.
Insertion:	Coronoid process and ramus of mandible.
Line of pull:	Anterior fibers: Vertical. Middle fibers: Diagonal. Posterior fibers: Horizontal.
Muscle action:	Bilaterally: Elevation and retrusion. Unilaterally: Ipsilateral lateral deviation.
Palpate:	On the lateral aspect of the skull above the TMJ.
Instructions to person:	While palpating bilaterally: Close your mouth. While palpating on the left: Move your jaw to the left.
MASSETER	One part is superficial and the other is deep; located in the posterior portion of the cheek between the mandibular angle and zygomatic arch.
	 FIGURE 13-16. Palpating the masseter.

(Continued...)

Sitting Postion *(continued)*

Position of person:	Mouth closed but jaw relaxed.
Origin:	Zygomatic arch of temporal bone and zygomatic process of maxilla.
Insertion:	Angle of ramus and coronoid process of mandible.
Line of pull:	Mostly vertical.
Muscle action:	Bilaterally: Elevation. Unilaterally: Ipsilateral lateral deviation.
Palpate:	Over the posterior part of the cheek below the zygomatic arch.
Instructions to person:	While palpating bilaterally or unilaterally: Clench and relax your jaw.
MEDIAL PTERYGOID	On the inside of the mandibular ramus.
Position of person:	Mouth open.
Origin:	Lateral pterygoid plate of the sphenoid bone and tuberosity of the maxilla.
Insertion:	Ramus and angle of the mandible.
Line of pull:	Diagonal.
Muscle action:	Bilaterally: Elevation, protrusion. Unilaterally: Contralateral lateral deviation.
Palpate:	Difficult but may possibly be palpated from inside the mouth. Wearing examination gloves, place your index finger inside the mouth and your thumb outside on the mandible. To distinguish from the masseter, have the person laterally deviate to the opposite side.
Instructions to person:	When palpating the right medial pterygoid say: "Move your jaw to the left."
LATERAL PTERYGOID	Deep.
Position of person:	Mouth closed.
Origin:	Lateral pterygoid plate and greater wing of the sphenoid.
Insertion:	Mandibular condyle and articular disk.
Line of pull:	Horizontal.
Muscle action:	Bilaterally: Depression, protrusion. Unilaterally: Contralateral lateral deviation.
Palpate:	Difficult but may possibly be palpated from inside the mouth. Wearing examination gloves, place your index finger inside the mouth behind the molars on the maxilla and your thumb outside in the same place. To distinguish from the masseter, have the person laterally deviate to the opposite side.
Instructions to person:	Open your mouth and move your jaw to the opposite side.

(Continued...)

SUPRAHYOIDS	Form a wall of muscles along the underside of the jaw between the mandible and the hyoid bone. All insert on the hyoid bone.
MYLOHYOID	Deep. Origin: Interior medial mandible.
GENIOHYOID	Deep. Origin: Mental spine of mandible.
STYLOHYOID	Deep: Origin: Styloid process of temporal bone.
Insertion:	All on the hyoid bone.
Muscle action:	Assists in depressing mandible.
Palpate:	Place your fingers along the underside of the mandible. Distinguishing between the individual suprahyoid muscles is difficult.
Instructions to person:	Press the tip of your tongue against the roof of your mouth.
DIGASTRIC	Deep.
Position of person:	Mouth closed.
Origin:	Anterior: Internal inferior mandible; Posterior: Mastoid process.
Insertion:	Hyoid.
Muscle action:	Assists in depressing mandible.
Palpate:	Place one finger on the mastoid process and another finger on the hyoid bone. Draw an imaginary line between the two points and place your fingers along this line. Place another finger under the person's chin.
Instructions to person:	Open your mouth against my finger.
INFRAHYOIDS	Located below the hyoid bone. For the TMJ, they serve to stabilize the hyoid so that the suprahyoid muscles can depress the mandible. All but the sternothyroid insert on the inferior border of the hyoid bone. The sternothyroid inserts on the thyroid cartilage.
STERNOHYOID	Deep. Origin: Medial end of clavicle, sternoclavicular ligament, manubrium of sternum.
STERNOTHYROID	Deep. Origin: Manubrium of sternum and cartilage of the first rib.
THYROHYOID	Deep. Origin: Thyroid cartilage.
OMOHYOID	Deep. Origin: Superior border of the scapula.
Muscle action:	Stabilizes the hyoid bone.
Palpate:	Difficult to distinguish between the sternohyoid and sternothyroid. Place your fingers along side the trachea just below the thyroid cartilage (Adam's apple) and medial to the sternocleidomastoid muscle. Use your other hand against the forehead to resist head and neck flexion.
Instructions to person:	Bring your chin to your chest.

7. People without proper head alignment often have difficulty swallowing. They may drool or choke when eating.

   With the head, neck, and trunk in the following three (3) positions, take a drink of water and eat a cracker or cookie. Use caution performing these activities. Make note of the ease of drinking and eating in each position.

   Position 1: With the head, neck, and upper trunk in proper alignment.

   Position 2: With the head, neck, and upper trunk in flexion.

   Position 3: With the head, neck, and upper trunk in hyperextension.

   A. In which position(s) was it easy to drink and eat?

   _____

   B. In which position(s) was it difficult to drink and eat?

   _____

   C. Explain.

   _____

8. Which motions of the TMJ do people typically use when chewing?

   _____

9. To bite off a piece of jerky requires which TMJ muscles to perform what type of contraction(s)?

   _____

10. An acrobat is hanging and spinning supported only by biting on a mouthpiece.
    A. Which TMJ motion(s) would definitely not be wanted?

    _____

    B. Which TMJ muscle(s) would prevent this unwanted motion?

    _____

■ ■ ■ Post-Lab Questions

Student's Name _____ Date Due _____

After you have completed the Worksheets and Lab Activities, answer the following questions without using your book or notes. When finished, check your answers.

1. For each muscle listed, check the motions for which the muscle is considered a prime mover.

Muscle	Elevation	Depression	Protrusion	Retrusion	Ipsilateral Lateral Deviation	Contralateral Lateral Deviation
Temporalis						
Masseter						
Medial pterygoid						
Lateral pterygoid						

2. What motions of the TMJ will be absent if cranial nerve V is severed?

_____

3. Describe the movement of the articular disk during left lateral deviation of the mandible.

_____

4. Bell's palsy is a condition resulting from insult to cranial nerve VII. The injury to the nerve is thought to occur as it exits a foramen in the mandible. Which TMJ muscles will be affected by an injury to cranial nerve VII?

_____

Neck and Trunk

Student's Name _____ Date Due _____

Complete the following questions prior to the lab class.

1. Define the following terms:

   Spine _____

   Facet _____

2. Indicate on Figure 14-1 the cervical, thoracic, lumbar, and sacral regions of the spine. Which of these regions are concave and which are convex anteriorly?

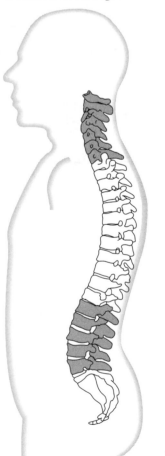

FIGURE 14-1. Vertebral column.

3. On Figures 14-2 through 14-7, label the following bones and landmarks:

BONES:	Occipital	Maxilla	Parietal
	Frontal	Mandible	Temporal
	Sphenoid	Zygomatic	

LANDMARKS:	Basilar area	Foramen magnum	Occipital condyles
	Mastoid process	External auditory meatus	

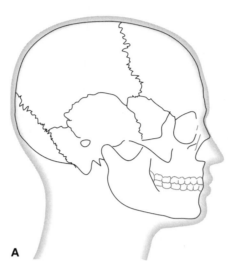
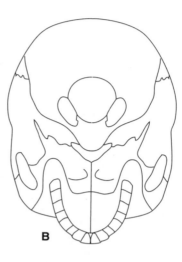

FIGURE 14-2. *(A)* and *(B)* Skull.

LANDMARKS ON VERTEBRA:	Body	Neural arch	Vertebral foramen
	Articular process	Pedicle	Lamina
	Transverse process	Spinous process	

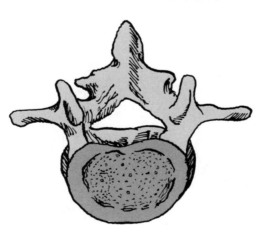

FIGURE 14-3. Vertebra.

Intervertebral foramen   Intervertebral disk   Facet joint

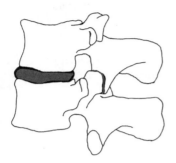

FIGURE 14-4. Vertebral joint.

ATLAS: Anterior arch   Posterior arch   Articular process
              Transverse process   Vertebral foramen   Transverse foramen

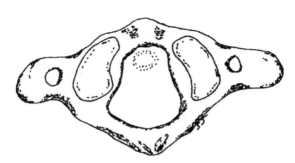

FIGURE 14-5. Superior view of the atlas.

AXIS: Dens   Transverse foramen   Superior articular process   Body
             Lamina   Spinous process   Transverse process

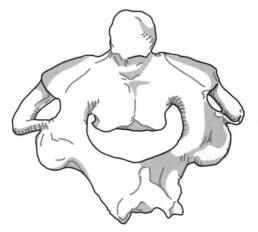

FIGURE 14-6. Posterior view of the axis.

Facets (3 shown)   Demifacet   Vertebral body
Spinous process   Rib

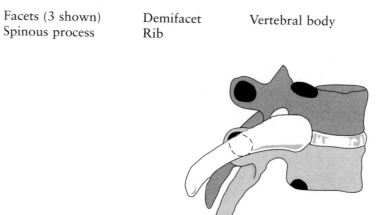

FIGURE 14-7. Thoracic vertebrae.

4. On Figure 14-8, label the following structures:

Body   Spinous process
Anterior longitudinal ligament   Posterior longitudinal ligament
Supraspinal ligament   Interspinal ligament
Ligamentum flavum   Lamina

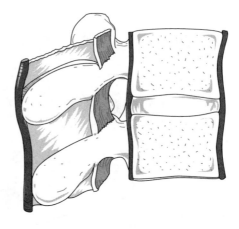

FIGURE 14-8. Vertebral parts and ligaments.

5. On Figures 14-9 through 14-13:
   A. Label the origin and insertion of the muscles listed.
   B. Join the origin and insertion to show the line of pull.

   Sternocleidomastoid

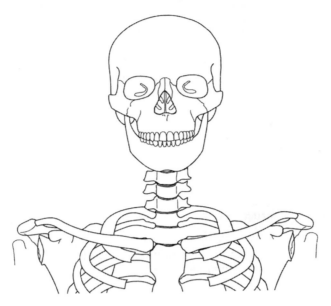

FIGURE 14-9. Sternocleidomastoid.

Splenius capitis   Splenius cervicis

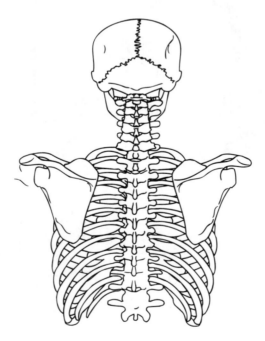

FIGURE 14-10. Splenius capitis and splenius cervicis.

Rectus abdominis   Transverse abdominis

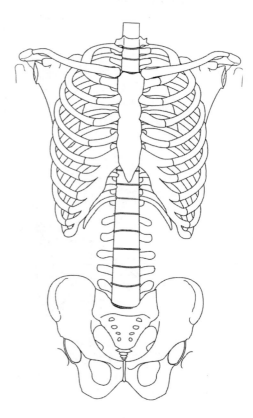

FIGURE 14-11. Rectus abdominis and transverse abdominis.

External oblique   Internal oblique

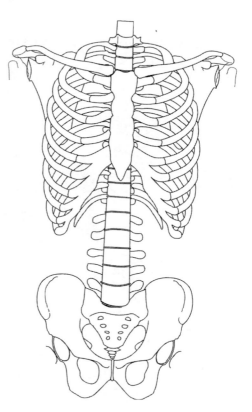

FIGURE 14-12. External oblique and internal oblique.

Quadratus lumborum
Erector spinae: Spinalis, longissimus, iliocostalis

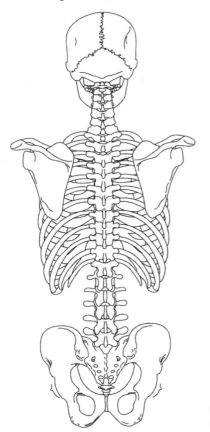

FIGURE 14-13. Quadratus lumborum and erector spinae: spinalis, longissimus, iliocostalis.

6. On Figure 14-4, label the three parts of the scalene muscle.

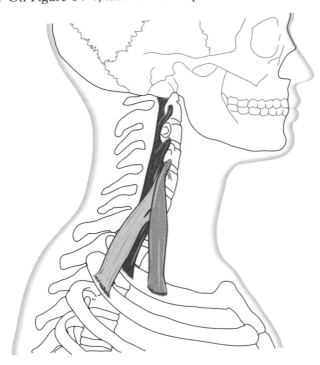

FIGURE 14-14. Scalenes.

7. For each of the following joints, give the indicated information:

Joint	Degrees of Freedom	Motions	Plane	Axis
Atlanto-occipital				
Atlantoaxial				

8. For the following joints, identify which surface is concave and which is convex.

Joint	Concave	Convex
Atlanto-occipital		
Atlantoaxial		

9. Facet joints are formed by the articulation between the _____ articular

processes of the vertebra below with the _____ articular processes
of the vertebra above.

10. What determines the extent, the type, and amount of motion possible at each part of the

vertebral column? _____

11. What limits spinal motion in the thoracic region?

_____

■ ■ ■ Lab Activities

Student's Name _____ Date Due _____

1. Perform the motions of the neck and trunk with your partner.
   A. Perform a motion and then your partner names the motion you performed.
   B. Your partner states a motion and you perform that motion.

2. Observe the amount of motion available at each joint in each plane. For each of the
   motions available, estimate the degrees of motion available and check the box that *most
   closely* describes that amount of motion. (Do not measure with a goniometer.)

Atlanto-occipital

Motions	0°–45°	46°–90°	91°–135°	136°–180°
Flexion				
Extension				

Atlantoaxial

Motions	0°–45°	46°–90°	91°–135°	136°–180°
Rotation to the right				
Rotation to the left				

3. Observe your partner flex, extend, laterally bend, and rotate. Indicate the amount of motion available in each of the three (3) regions of the spinal column as minimal or maximum.

Spinal Region	Flexion/Extension	Lateral Bending	Rotation
Cervical			
Thoracic			
Lumbar			

4. On the skeleton, anatomical models, and at least one partner, locate, palpate, and observe the following structures. Most of these structures cannot be palpated. The reference position is the anatomical position. Having pictures for reference is helpful when trying to find structures.

Skull

Occipital bone or Occiput	Posterior inferior part of the skull. The area above the occipital protuberance is superficial. The part below curves in under the head and is covered by muscles. Putting your hand on the back of your head covers much of the occiput. FIGURE 14-15. Palpating the occiput.
Occipital protuberance	The small prominence in the center of the occiput. Palpate over the skull in the midline of the occiput.
Basilar area	Base, or inferior, portion of the occiput. Cannot be palpated.
Foramen magnum	Opening in the occipital bone through which the spinal cord enters the cranium. Cannot be palpated.
Occipital condyles	Located laterally to the foramen magnum on the occiput; articulates with atlas. Cannot be palpated.

(Continued...)

Temporal bone	Forms part of the base and lateral inferior sides of the cranium. Palpate on the side of the head just anterior and superior to the ear.
Mastoid process	Bony prominence behind the ear lobe; attachment for the sternocleidomastoid. Palpate just behind the ear.

Vertebrae

Body	Anterior portion of the vertebra; C1 and 2 do not have a body. Cannot be palpated.
Neural arch or Vertebral arch	Posterior portion of the vertebra. Cannot be palpated. Only the transverse and spinous processes can be palpated. See later.
Vertebral foramen	Opening formed by the joining of the body and neural arch through which the spinal cord passes. Cannot be palpated.
Pedicle	Portion of the neural arch posterior to the body and anterior to the lamina. Cannot be palpated.
Lamina	Posterior portion of the neural arch that unites from each side of the midline. Cannot be palpated.
Transverse process	Formed at the union of the lamina and pedicle, the lateral projections of the arch to which muscles and ligaments attach. Palpate on the lateral aspect of the neck inferior to the ear lobes. **FIGURE 14-16.** Cervical transverse processes.
Vertebral notches	Depressions located on the superior and inferior surfaces of the pedicle. Cannot be palpated.
Intervertebral foramen	Opening formed by the superior notch of the vertebra below and the inferior notch of the vertebra above. Cannot be palpated.
Articular process	Projecting superiorly and inferiorly off the posterior surface of each lamina. Superior articular processes face posteriorly or medially whereas inferior processes face anteriorly or laterally. Cannot be palpated.
Spinous process	Most posterior projection on the neural arch; located at the junction of the two laminae. It is the attachment for many muscles and ligaments. The tips of spinous processes can be palpated as a ridge in the midline of the back. In the cervical area, the spinous processes can be palpated under the ligamentum nuchae when the neck is in hyperextension. The spinous processes can also be palpated in the thoracic and lumbar regions.

(Continued...)

Intervertebral Disk

Annulus fibrosus	The outer portion of the disk consisting of several concentrically arranged fibrocartilaginous rings. Cannot be palpated.
Nucleus pulposus	Pulpy gelatinous substance with high water content in the center of the disk. Cannot be palpated.

Atlas

Atlas C1	The first cervical vertebra upon which the cranium rests. Round without a body or a spinous process. Cannot be palpated on most people.
Anterior arch	The anterior portion of the atlas. Cannot be palpated.

Axis

Axis C2	Second cervical vertebra. The transverse and spinous processes can be palpated on the side and posterior midline respectively.
Dens or Odontoid process	Large vertical projection located anteriorly on the axis. Cannot be palpated.

Other Structures

C7 or Vertebra prominens	Has a long and prominent spinous process. Easily palpated, and often quite visible, with neck flexion.

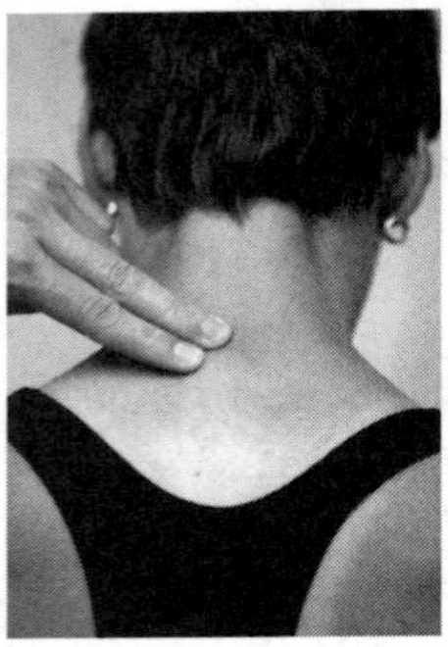

FIGURE 14-17. Palpating C7.

Transverse foramen	Holes in the transverse process of the cervical vertebra through which the vertebral artery passes. Cannot be palpated.
Facet or costal facets	Located superiorly and inferiorly on the sides of the bodies and on the transverse processes of the thoracic vertebrae. Articulates with ribs. Cannot be palpated.
Demifacet	Partial or half facet; located laterally on the superior and inferior edges of the vertebral body where ribs articulate with the thoracic vertebrae. Cannot be palpated.

(Continued...)

5. Using a skeleton or model of the spinal column locate where each of the following joints and ligaments are located.

Atlanto-occipital joint	Joint of the 1st cervical vertebra and occiput. Cannot be palpated.
Atlantoaxial joints	Joint between C1 and C2. Cannot be palpated.
Median atlantoaxial joints	Synovial articulation between the dens (odontoid) process of the axis and the anterior arch of the atlas anteriorly and the transverse ligament posteriorly. Cannot be palpated.
Lateral atlantoaxial joints	Joints between the articular processes of two vertebrae. Cannot be palpated.
Facet joints	Articulations on posterior and lateral aspects of the vertebrae; the superior articular process of the vertebra below and the inferior articular process of the vertebra above. Cannot be palpated.
Anterior longitudinal ligament	Located on the anterior surface of the bodies of the vertebral column. Cannot be palpated.
Posterior longitudinal ligament	Located on the posterior surface of the vertebral bodies in the vertebral foramen. Cannot be palpated.
Supraspinal ligament	Located on the posterior along the tips of the spinous processes extending from C7 to sacrum. Palpate by placing finger tips between two adjacent thoracic or lumbar spinous processes and having the person slightly flex the trunk. This movement causes the ligament to become taut.
Ligamentum nuchae or nuchal ligament	Located on the posterior along the tips of the spinous processes in the cervical region. Palpate by placing finger tips between two adjacent cervical spinous processes and having the person slightly flex the neck. This movement causes the ligament to become taut. 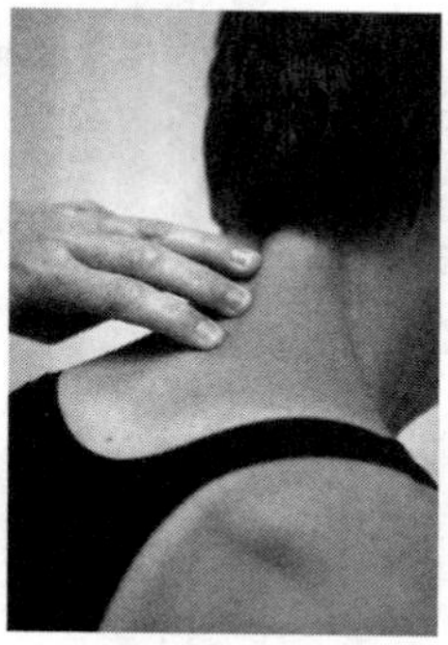 **FIGURE 14-18.** Palpating the nuchal ligament.
Interspinal ligament	Joins the spinous processes of adjunct vertebrae. Cannot be palpated.
Ligamentum flavum	Located on the anterior surface of the neural arch inside the vertebral foramen. Cannot be palpated

6. On the skeleton, anatomical models, and at least one partner:

   A. Locate the origin and insertion of the muscle on the skeleton.

   B. Stretch a large rubber band taut by placing one end at the origin and the other end at the insertion of a muscle on the skeleton.

   C. Perform the motion that the muscle does and observe how the rubber band becomes less taut and shorter, similar to the muscle shortening as it contracts.

   D. Perform the opposite motion and observe how the rubber band becomes tauter and longer, similar to the muscle lengthening as it is being stretched.

   E. After locating the muscle on the skeleton, locate the muscle on your partner. The position described for locating the muscle on your partner is the manual muscle test position for a fair or better grade of muscle strength. Not all origins, insertions, and muscle bellies can be palpated on your partner.

   F. When possible, palpate the origin, insertion, and muscle belly of each muscle by:

      1) Placing your fingers on the origin and insertion, and asking your partner to contract the muscle.

      2) Moving your fingers from the origin and insertion over the contracting muscle.

      3) Asking your partner to relax the muscle and again moving your fingers from the origin to the insertion over the muscle.

      4) Note the difference between the contracting and relaxed muscle.

   G. In the following tables, the information needed to palpate each muscle is provided. The information includes position of the person, origin and insertion of the muscle, the line of pull of the muscle, the muscle's action, instructions to give to the person to make the muscle contract, and, finally, information on the best location to palpate the muscle.

Supine Position

STERNOCLEIDOMASTOID	Located superficially on anterior aspect of neck.
	FIGURE 14-19. Palpating the sternocleidomastoid muscle. FIGURE 14-20. Palpating both sternocleidomastoid muscles.
Position of person:	Unilateral: Head turned to one side. Bilateral: Head in midline.
Origin:	Sternum and clavicle.
Insertion:	Mastoid process.
Line of pull:	Diagonal.

(Continued...)

Muscle action:	Unilaterally: Laterally bends neck; rotates head to opposite side. Bilaterally: Flexes head and neck; hyperextends head.
Palpate:	Anterior aspect of neck between the sternal end of the clavicle and the mastoid process.
Instructions to person:	Unilaterally: Looking to the side, lift your head off the table. Bilaterally: Looking ahead, lift your head off the table.

SCALENES	Deep on lateral aspect of neck. 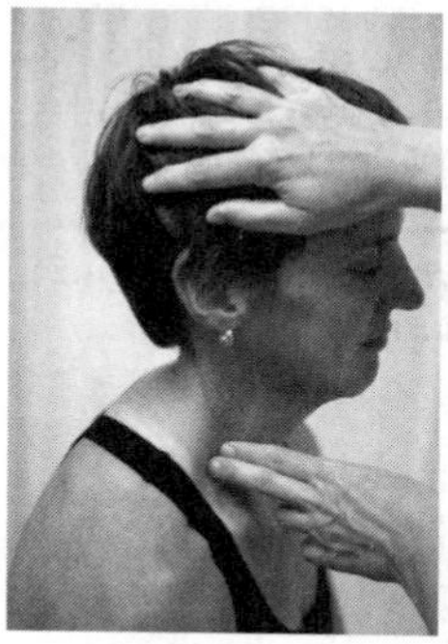 **FIGURE 14-21.** Palpating the right scalene muscles.
Position of person:	Head in the midline.
Origin:	Anterior scalene: Transverse processes of C3–C6. Middle scalene: Transverse processes of C2–C7. Posterior scalene: Transverse processes of C5–C7.
Insertion:	Anterior scalene: Superior surface of the 1st rib. Middle scalene: Superior surface of the 1st rib. Posterior scalene: Second rib.
Line of pull:	Vertical.
Muscle action:	Unilaterally: Laterally bends neck. Bilaterally: Assists with neck flexion.
Palpate:	On lateral aspect of neck between the sternocleidomastoid and the erector spinae.
Instructions to person:	Unilaterally: Move your ear toward your shoulder. Bilaterally: Lift your head off the table.

RECTUS ABDOMINIS	Located superficially on abdomen. 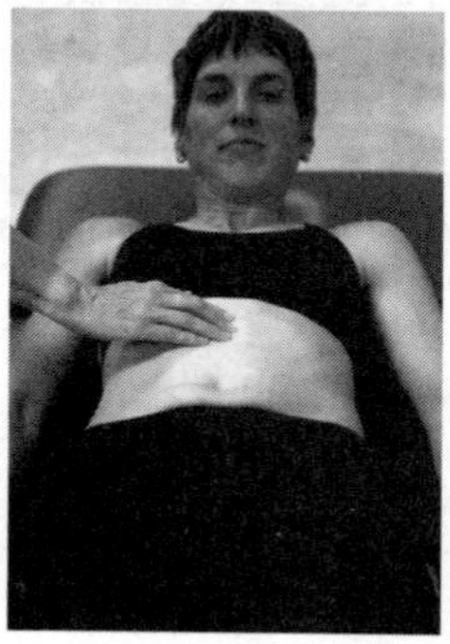 **FIGURE 14-22.** Palpating the rectus abdominis muscle.

(Continued...)

Supine Position *(continued)*

Position of person:	Arms at sides.
Origin:	Pubis.
Insertion:	Costal cartilages of 5th, 6th, and 7th ribs.
Line of pull:	Vertical on the anterior trunk.
Muscle action:	Trunk flexion.
Palpate:	Midline of abdomen.
Instructions to person:	Curl your body until your scapula are off the table.

EXTERNAL OBLIQUE	Located superficially on lateral aspect of abdomen.

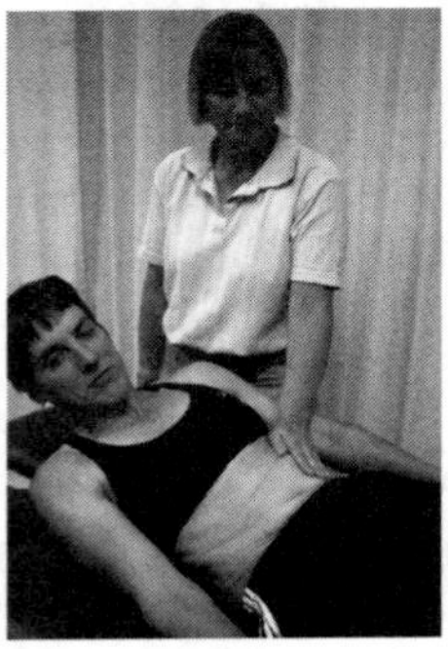

FIGURE 14-23. Palpating the left external oblique muscle.

Position of person:	Arms at sides.
Origin:	Lower 8th ribs laterally.
Insertion:	Iliac crest and linea alba.
Line of pull:	Diagonal on the anterior trunk.
Muscle action:	Unilaterally: Lateral bending; rotation to opposite side. Bilaterally: Trunk flexion; compression of abdomen.
Palpate:	On the left lateral abdomen for left external oblique muscle.
Instructions to person:	To examine the left external oblique: Reach toward your right hip lifting your left shoulder off the table.

INTERNAL OBLIQUE	Located deep to external oblique muscle.
Position of person:	Arms at sides.
Origin:	Inguinal ligament, iliac crest, thoracolumbar fascia.
Insertion:	10th, 11th, and 12th ribs, abdominal aponeurosis.
Line of pull:	Diagonal on the anterior trunk.

(Continued...)

Muscle action:	Unilaterally: Lateral bending; rotation to same side. Bilaterally: Trunk flexion; compression of the abdomen.
Palpate:	On left lateral abdomen for left internal oblique muscle, deep to the left external oblique.
Instructions to person:	To examine the left internal oblique: Reach toward your left hip lifting your right shoulder off the table (left external oblique is not contracting during this motion).
TRANSVERSE ABDOMINIS	Deep to the oblique muscles.
Position of person:	Arms at sides.
Origin:	Inguinal ligament, iliac crest, thoracolumbar fascia, and last six ribs.
Insertion:	Abdominal aponeurosis and linea alba.
Line of pull:	Horizontal on the anterior trunk.
Muscle action:	Compression of abdomen.
Palpate:	Lateral aspect of abdomen. Cannot be differentiated from other more superficial anterior trunk muscles.
Instructions to person:	Cough.
PREVERTEBRAL	Deep on anterior aspect of neck.
Position of person:	Head in midline.
Origin:	Collectively, from bodies and transverse processes of upper cervical vertebra.
Insertion:	Collectively, to occipital bone and transverse processes and bodies of upper cervical vertebra.
Line of pull:	Vertical on the anterior trunk.
Muscle action:	Flex head on C1.
Palpate:	Cannot be palpated.
Instruction to observe muscle action:	Tuck your chin.
QUADRATUS LUMBORUS	Deep.
Position of person:	Good postural alignment.
Origin:	Iliac crest.
Insertion:	12th rib, transverse processes of all five lumbar vertebrae.
Line of pull:	Vertical on the lateral side of the trunk.

(Continued...)

Supine Position *(continued)*

Muscle action:	Trunk lateral bending; hip hiking (elevation of one side of the pelvis).
Palpate:	Difficult to palpate. Maybe possible on a thin person by palpating very deep on the lateral side of the torso between the lower ribs and the iliac crest.
Instructions to person:	Slide the left side of your pelvis toward your left shoulder keeping your pelvis on the table.

Prone Position

ERECTOR SPINAE	Located along the vertebral column, some are deep and some are superficial.

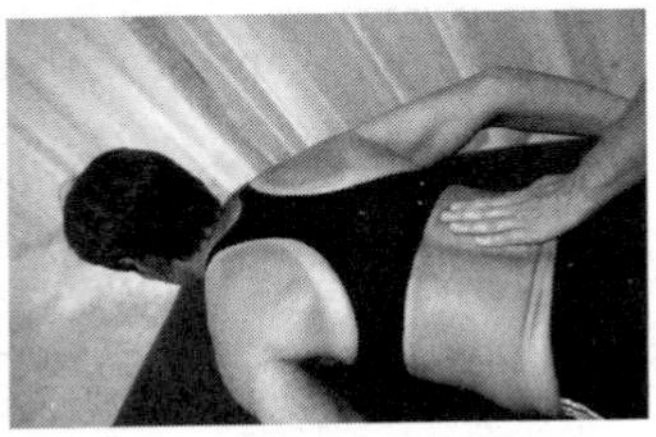

FIGURE 14-24. Palpating the erector spinae muscle.

Position of person:	Head in midline, shoulders parallel to the pelvis.
Origin:	Spinalis group: Nuchal ligament and spinous processes of cervical and thoracic vertebrae. Longissimus group: Transverse processes from occiput to sacrum. Iliocostalis group: Sacrum, ilium, and ribs.
Insertion:	Spinalis group: Occiput and transverse processes. Longissimus group: Transverse processes and adjacent ribs. Iliocostalis group: Transverse processes to C7 and the ribs.
Line of pull:	Vertical.
Muscle action:	Unilaterally: Lateral bending. Bilaterally: Extend neck and trunk.
Palpate:	Posterior neck and trunk: Spinalis medial, iliocostalis lateral, longissimus between the other two. Difficult to differentiate.
Instructions to person:	Unilaterally: Move your ear toward your shoulder. Bilaterally: Lift your head off the table.
TRANSVERSOSPINALIS	Posterior, deep to erector spinae. Three muscles: Semispinalis, multifidus, rotators.
Position of person:	Head in midline, shoulders parallel to the pelvis.
Origin:	Transverse processes.
Insertion:	Spinous processes of vertebra above.
Line of pull:	Diagonal on the posterior side of the trunk.

(Continued...)

Muscle action:	Unilaterally: Rotation to opposite side.
	Bilaterally: Extend trunk.
Palpate:	Cannot be palpated.
Instruction to observe muscle action:	Unilaterally: To examine the left muscles: Raise your head and right shoulder off the table.
	Bilaterally: Look up and lift your head and trunk off the table.
INTERSPINALES AND INTERTRANSVERSARII	Posterior, deep to erector spinae.
Position of person:	Head in midline, shoulders parallel to the pelvis.
Origin:	Interspinales: Spinous process below.
	Intertransversarii: Transverse process below.
Insertion:	Interspinales: Spinous process above.
	Intertransversarii: Transverse process above.
Line of pull:	Vertical on the posterior side of the trunk.
Muscle action:	Unilaterally: Lateral bending.
	Bilaterally: Extend trunk.
Palpate:	Cannot be palpated.
Instruction to observe muscle action:	Unilaterally: Slide your left shoulder toward your left pelvis keeping your trunk on the table.
	Bilaterally: Look up and lift your head and trunk off the table.

7. Perform the following two variations of sit-ups. Sit up only until scapula clear the table. Start with the arms at the side reaching forward as the sit-up is performed.

   A. With hips and knees flexed so feet are close to buttocks.

   B. With legs extended.

   How does hip position make a difference in performance of a sit-up?

   _____

   _____

8. Perform the following three variations of a sit-up to determine which is the easiest and which is the hardest? Explain why?

   A. Hands overhead.

   B. Hands crossed over chest.

   C. Arms extended in front.

   _____

   _____

9. Perform trunk flexion (trunk curl) in supine. Compare the range of trunk motion achieved with the range of motion achieved in questions 7 and 8.

A. Where does the additional ROM come from in the sit-up exercises in questions 7 and 8?

_____

B. Which method, sit-up or trunk curl, is less likely to increase lumbar lordosis?

_____ Sit up   _____ Trunk curl

10. With your partner lying on a table with hands on shoulders and legs extended, place one of your hands under your partner's lower lumbar region. Place your other hand on your partner's abdomen. Ask your partner to press the low back into the table. Complete the following:

A.

Motion Performed	Agonist	Antagonist

B. If your partner is unable to press the low back into the table, which muscles may be too short to permit the movement to occur?

_____

C. If your partner is unable to press the low back into the table, which muscles may be too weak or long to perform the movement?

_____

11. In the standing position, slide your left hand down the side of your leg, thereby bringing your shoulder closer to your knee.

A. What motion did you perform? _____

B. Which muscle(s) performed the motion? _____

C. What type of contraction has the agonist performed?

_____ Eccentric   _____ Concentric

■ ■ ■ Post-Lab Questions

Student's Name _____ Date Due _____

After you have completed the Worksheets and Lab Activities, answer the following questions without using your book or notes. When finished, check your answers.

1. List the other terms used to describe the following bones or landmarks:

A. Dens: _____

B. Seventh cervical vertebra: _____

C. First cervical vertebra: _____

D. Second cervical vertebra: _____

E. Neural arch: _____

2. Which vertebra does not have a spinous process or a body? _____

3. C1 articulates with which landmark of the skull? _____

4. What position does the head assume when the left sternocleidomastoid performs a concentric contraction?

      _____ Lateral bending with rotation   _____ Lateral bending with rotation
              to the right   to the left

5. Which oblique muscles perform a sit up with rotation to the right?

      _____ Right internal and left external   _____ Left internal and right external
              oblique   oblique

6. When performing bilateral leg raises, which muscle group must perform what type of contraction to prevent the low back from arching?

_____

7. What muscle groups make up the erector spinae muscle group?

_____

Respiratory System

■ ■ ■ Worksheets

Student's Name _____ Date Due _____

Complete the following questions prior to lab class.

1. Match the following phases of respiration with the appropriate definition.

    _____ Quiet inspiration   A. Muscles compress the abdomen

    _____ Deep inspiration   B. Mostly a passive action

    _____ Forced inspiration   C. Uses muscles that pull up ribs

    _____ Quiet expiration   D. Diaphragm and external intercostals are prime movers

    _____ Forced expiration   E. In a state of "air hunger"

2. Describe the differences between diaphragmatic breathing and chest breathing in terms of energy required and amount of air exchanged.

    _____

    _____

3. A. What is a Valsalva maneuver?

    _____

    B. When do people tend to use the Valsalva maneuver?

    _____

    C. Describe the series of events that have the potential to cause cardiac disturbance when a person performs a Valsalva maneuver.

    _____

    _____

4. List the anatomical structures that are referred to as the "bronchial tree."

    _____

5. On Figure 15-1, label the following joints, bones and landmarks:

    True ribs   False ribs   Floating ribs   Costal cartilage
      Manubrium   Xiphoid process   Sternal body

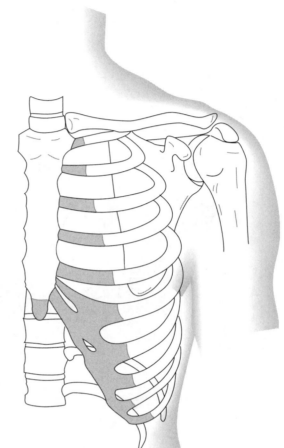

FIGURE 15-1. Rib cage.

6. On Figure 15-2:

    A. Label the joints and bones:

        Costovertebral joints   Vertebral body   Rib   Transverse process

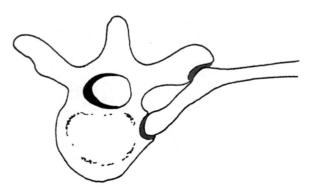

FIGURE 15-2. Costovertebral joint.

B. Identify the following respiratory structures on Figure 15-3:

Larynx Trachea Bronchioles Alveoli
Nasal cavity Oral cavity Nasopharynx Oral pharynx
Diaphragm Laryngopharynx Mediastinum Bronchii

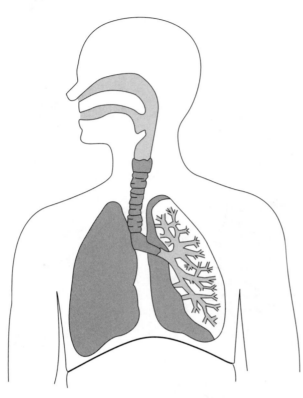

FIGURE 15-3. Respiratory structures.

7. On Figure 15-4:
   A. Label the origin and insertion of the muscles listed.
   B. Join the origin and insertion to show the line of pull.

   Diaphragm External intercostal Internal intercostal

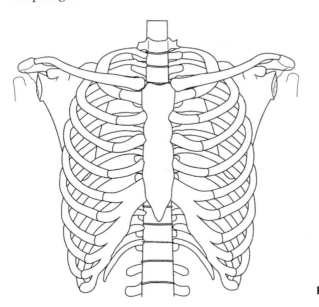

FIGURE 15-4. Rib cage.

8. At the following joint, identify which surface is concave and which is convex.

Joint	Concave	Convex
Costovertebral		

9. Check the column that indicates the movement of the ribs associated with each phase of respiration.

Phase of Respiration	Elevation	Depression
Inspiration		
Expiration		

10. Describe the function of the soft palate.

_____

11. List the three parts of the pharynx.

_____

12. During inspiration air flows _____ the lungs because the rib cage _____.

During expiration air flows _____ the lungs because the rib cage _____.

13. List the accessory muscles of respiration:

Inspiration	Expiration

■ ■ ■ Lab Activities

Student's Name _____ Date Due _____

1. Observe the amount of motion available as the rib cage moves during quiet respiration and during deep respiration. Use a tape measure to measure the difference in rib cage circumference. Compare the measurements of classmates, who volunteer to participate, to determine any differences based on gender, age, and smoker/nonsmoker.

2. On the skeleton, anatomical models, and at least one partner, locate, palpate, and observe the following structures. The reference position is the anatomical position. Having pictures for reference is helpful when trying to find structures. Not all structures can be palpated on your partner.

Rib Cage	All of the ribs and sternum
True ribs	The upper seven ribs. The 1st rib is difficult to palpate. Palpate posterior to the clavicle through the scalene muscles.
False ribs	Ribs 8–10 attach indirectly to sternum via costal cartilage of the 7th rib. Palpate on the lateral chest wall.
Floating ribs	Ribs 11–12 have no anterior attachment. Palpate the lateral ends on a person in the prone position. Reach across the person's body to the opposite chest wall. Move your hand inferiorly to the bottom of the rib cage and press deep into soft tissue. The floating ribs are deep to the erector spinae muscles.
Sternum	Palpate on the midline of the anterior chest wall.
Sternal notch	Superior border of sternum between the sternal ends of the clavicles. Palpate between the clavicles at the proximal end of the sternum. See Chapter 8.
Manubrium	Superior portion of the sternum. As a landmark, it articulates with the clavicle and the first two ribs. Palpate between the sternal notch and body of the sternum. See Chapter 8.
Body of sternum	Middle portion of the sternum. Palpate between the manubrium and xiphoid process. See Chapter 8.
Xiphoid process	Inferior tip of the sternum. Palpate at the distal end of the sternum. See Chapter 8.
Costovertebral joints	Articulation of the vertebra and ribs. Cannot be palpated.
Sternocostal joints	Articulation of the sternum and ribs. Difficult to distinguish.
Costal cartilage	Cartilage joining ribs and sternum. Difficult to distinguish.

3. On a skeleton, anatomical models, and at least one partner:
   A. Locate the origin and insertion of the muscle on the skeleton.
   B. Stretch a large rubber band taut by placing one end at the origin and the other end at the insertion of a muscle on the skeleton.

C. Perform the motion that the muscle does and observe how the rubber band becomes less taut and shorter, similar to the muscle shortening as it contracts.

D. Perform the opposite motion and observe how the rubber band becomes tauter and longer, similar to the muscle lengthening as it is being stretched.

E. After locating the muscle on the skeleton, locate the muscle on your partner. The position described for locating the muscle on your partner is the manual muscle test position for a fair or better grade of muscle strength. Not all origins, insertions, and muscle bellies can be palpated on your partner.

F. When possible, palpate the origin, insertion, and muscle belly of each muscle by:

1) Placing your fingers on the origin and insertion, and asking your partner to contract the muscle.

2) Moving your fingers from the origin and insertion over the contracting muscle.

3) Asking your partner to relax the muscle and again moving your fingers from the origin to the insertion over the muscle.

4) Note the difference between the contracting and relaxed muscle.

G. In the following tables, the information needed to palpate each muscle is provided. The information includes position of the person, origin and insertion of the muscle, the line of pull of the muscle, the muscle's action, instructions to give to the person to make the muscle contract, and, finally, information on the best location to palpate the muscle.

Supine Position

DIAPHRAGM	Located deep, separates thoracic and abdominal cavities.
	FIGURE 15-5. Palpating the diaphragm.
Position of person:	Quiet breathing.
Origin:	Xiphoid process, lower six ribs, upper lumbar vertebrae.
Insertion:	Central tendon.
Line of pull:	Diagonal.
Muscle action:	Inspiration.
Observe:	Chest and abdomen rise.
Palpate:	Palpate by curling your fingers under the inferior edge of the rib cage bilaterally. You may not feel the contraction of the diaphragm but other tissues being pushed out as the diaphragm contracts. Alternatively, place your hand over the upper abdomen noting the rise and fall of the abdomen as the person breathes.
Instructions to person:	Breathe in and out at your normal rate.

(Continued...)

Supine Position (continued)

EXTERNAL INTERCOSTALS	Located between ribs. **FIGURE 15-6.** Palpating the external intercostals.
Position of person:	Quiet breathing.
Origin:	Rib above.
Insertion:	Rib below.
Line of pull:	Diagonal.
Muscle action:	Elevate ribs.
Palpate:	Between adjacent ribs on the side of the rib cage, inferior to the pectoralis major muscle attachments.
Instructions to person:	Breathe in and out at your normal rate.
INTERNAL INTERCOSTALS	Located between ribs deep to external intercostals.
Position of person:	Quiet breathing.
Origin:	Rib below.
Insertion:	Rib above.
Line of pull:	Diagonal.
Muscle action:	Depress ribs.
Palpate:	Between adjacent ribs; difficult as they are deep muscles and difficult to distinguish from the external intercostals.
Instructions to person:	Breathe in and out at your normal rate.

4. Using two pencils and the skeleton, align both pencils, with lead end pointing up, on the anterior of the rib cage in the direction of the muscle fibers of the external intercostal muscles. Move one pencil around the ribs to the posterior rib cage. Compare the alignment of the pencils.

   A. Anteriorly, is the eraser end pointing _____ medially or _____ laterally?

   B. Posteriorly, is the eraser end pointing _____ medially or _____ laterally?

   C. Why does the angle appear to change?

   _____

5. During quiet inspiration the diaphragm is contracting:

   _____ Concentrically   _____ Eccentrically   _____ Isometrically

6. Palpate your partner's upper trapezius and sternocleidomastoid muscles during quiet breathing and as your partner takes deep breaths. Is there any difference? Why?

_____

7. What positions of the upper extremities do speed runners often assume immediately after a race? Why?

_____

_____

8. Persons with chronic obstructive respiratory disease often sit leaning forward propped on their arms. How does this posture contribute to ease of respiration?

_____

_____

9. Why might a person with emphysema lean with the forearms on the handgrip of a grocery cart while walking through a grocery store?

_____

10. With your partner in the supine position, head on a small pillow, and legs supported so the low back is relaxed:

   A. Palpate your partner's rib cage and abdomen during quiet breathing. What movement do you see and feel?

   _____

   B. Palpate your partner's upper and lower rib cage during quiet breathing. What movement do you see and feel?

   _____

   C. Repeat A and B as you partner takes deep breaths. Describe any changes and explain why they occur.

   _____

   _____

   D. Palpate your partner's rib cage and abdomen as your partner coughs, sneezes, and talks. Compare and contrast the movements of the rib cage and abdomen during these maneuvers and to movements during quiet respiration.

   _____

   _____

11. In many sports as athletes perform a strenuous activity, such as during the lift for a power lifter, throwing the shot-put, or returning a serve, they can be heard to exhale. Why is this advantageous?

_____

■ ■ ■ Post-Lab Questions

Student's Name _____ Date Due _____

After you have completed the Worksheets and Lab Activities, answer the following questions without using your book or notes. When finished, check your answers.

1. List the bones of the rib cage.

   _____

2. List the joints of the rib cage.

   _____

3. List the motions of the rib cage.

   _____

4. List the muscles of quiet respiration.

   _____

5. What is the function of the upper trapezius during respiration by persons with chronic obstructive respiratory disease?

   _____

6. What is the innervation of the prime movers for respiration?

   _____

7. Cervical spinal cord lesions can interfere with the ability of individuals to breathe on their own. Above what level of spinal cord lesion does an individual require assistance of a ventilator to breathe?

   _____

Pelvic Girdle

■ ■ ■ Worksheets

Student's Name _____ Date Due _____

Complete the following questions prior to the lab class.

1. Match the following terms with the appropriate definition:

———— False pelvis

———— Pelvic inlet

———— Pelvic outlet

———— True pelvis

———— Pelvic cavity

———— Nutation

———— Counternutation

A. Sacral base moves anteriorly and inferiorly

B. A line from the tip of the coccyx to the inferior surface of the pubic symphysis

C. Occurs when the base of the sacrum moves posteriorly and superiorly

D. Bony area between the iliac crests and superior to the pelvic inlet.

E. Located between the inlet and the outlet of the pelvis

F. Located between the sacral promontory and superior border of symphysis pubis

G. Forms the birth canal

2. On Figures 16-1A, B, and C, label the following bones, landmarks, and joints of the pelvic girdle:

BONES AND LANDMARKS

A. Sacrum:

Base   Superior articular process   Auricular surface
Posterior foramina   Ala

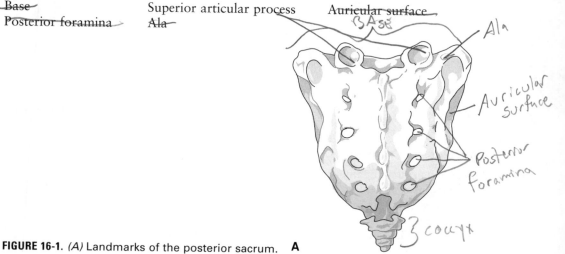

FIGURE 16-1. *(A)* Landmarks of the posterior sacrum. **A**

B. HIP BONES: Ilium   Ischium   Pubis
   LANDMARKS: Iliac crest   Greater sciatic notch   Ischial tuberosity
                 PSIS   PIIS   Ischial body
                 Ischial spine   ASIS   Lesser sciatic notch
                 AIIS   Acetabulum   Superior ramus
                 Body of pubis   Inferior ramus

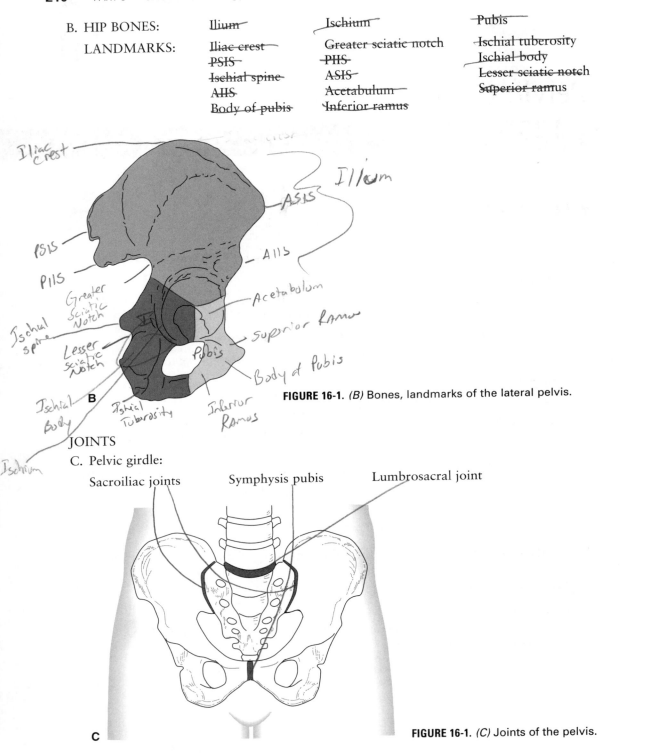

FIGURE 16-1. *(B)* Bones, landmarks of the lateral pelvis.

JOINTS

C. Pelvic girdle:

Sacroiliac joints   Symphysis pubis   Lumbrosacral joint

FIGURE 16-1. *(C)* Joints of the pelvis.

3. On Figures 16-2A, B, and C, label the following ligaments:

   Anterior sacroiliac ligament
   Short posterior sacroiliac ligament   Long posterior sacroiliac ligament
   Sacrotuberous ligament   Sacrospinous ligament
   Iliolumbar ligament   Superior pubic ligament
   Inferior pubic ligament   Lumbrosacral ligament
   Inguinal ligament

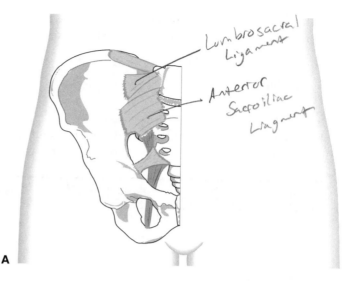

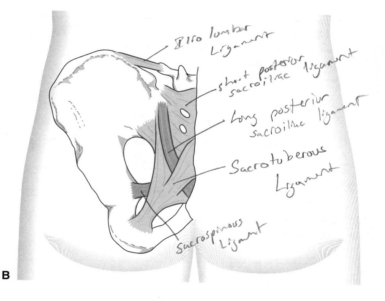

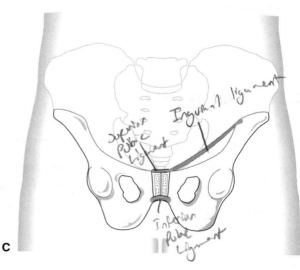

FIGURE 16-2. *(A)* Ligaments of the anterior pelvis, *(B)* ligaments of the posterior pelvis, and (C) ligaments of the pubic symphysis.

4. Indicate which of the following statements are true of the female pelvis and which are true of the male pelvis by placing an F or M respectively by the statement.

_____ Heart-shaped pelvic cavity opening   _____ Rounded pelvic cavity opening

_____ Short pelvic cavity   _____ Funnel-shaped pelvic cavity

_____ Short sacrum   _____ Ischial tuberosities far apart

5. For the following joint, indicate which motions are available, in which plane the motion occurs, and about which axis the motion occurs.

Joint	Motions	Plane	Axis
Sacroiliac			

6. List the trunk and hip motions that accompany SI joint motions.

SI Motion	Trunk	Hip
Nutation (flexion)		
Counternutation (extension)		

7. Review previous chapters and list the anterior trunk muscles that attach to the pelvis.

_____

_____

8. Review previous chapters and list the posterior trunk and upper extremity muscles that attach to the pelvis.

_____

_____

9. List three motions of the pelvis.

_____   _____   _____

■ ■ ■ Lab Activities

Student's Name _____ Date Due _____

1. Perform the motions of the pelvis (lateral, anterior, and posterior tilt, and rotation).
   A. Perform a motion and then your partner names the motion you performed.
   B. Your partner states a motion and then you perform that motion.

2. As you perform the following pelvic motions, what happens at the lumbar spine and hip?

Pelvic Motion	Vertebral Spine	Hip
Anterior pelvic tilt		
Posterior pelvic tilt		
Lateral pelvic tilt to the right		

3. For each of the motions of the pelvis:
   A. Place your open left hand in the correct orientation to represent the plane of a motion.
   B. Place your right index finger to indicate the axis of that motion.
   C. Enter the plane and axis for each motion in the following chart.

Pelvic Motions	Plane	Axis
Anterior/posterior tilt		
Lateral tilt		
Rotation		

4. On the skeleton, anatomical models, and at least one partner, locate, palpate, and observe the following structures. The reference position is the anatomical position. Having pictures for reference is helpful when trying to find structures. Not all structures can be palpated on your partner.

Sacrum

Base	Superior surface of S1. Cannot be palpated.
Promontory	Ridge projecting along the anterior edge of the body of S1. Cannot be palpated.
Superior articular process	Located posteriorly on the base, it articulates with the inferior articular process of L5. Cannot be palpated.
Ala	Lateral flared wings that are actually fused transverse processes. Cannot be palpated.
Foramina	Four pair located on the anterior and dorsal surfaces lateral to midline. They serve as the exit for the anterior and posterior divisions of the sacral nerves. The anterior foramina are larger and cannot be palpated. Difficult to palpate on posterior surface.
Auricular surface	Located on the lateral surface of the sacrum and articulates with the ilium. Cannot be palpated.
Pelvic surface	Concave anterior surface. Cannot be palpated.

Ilium

Tuberosity	Large roughened area between the posterior portion of the iliac crest and the auricular surface. It is the attachment for the interosseous ligament. Cannot be palpated.
Auricular surface	The articular surface of the ilium with the sacrum. Located inferior and anterior to the iliac tuberosity. Cannot be palpated.
Iliac crest	Superior margin of ilium extending from the ASIS to the PSIS. Iliac crests appear to be located more superiorly in men than women. Palpate by placing your hand on the top margin of the pelvis (place your hands on your hips).
Posterior superior iliac spine (PSIS)	Posterior projection of the iliac crest. It is the attachment for the posterior sacroiliac ligaments. Palpate by placing your hand on the iliac crest and moving posterior and medially to the first protuberance. A "dimple" is usually observable over the PSIS.
Posterior inferior iliac spine (PIIS)	Protuberance located inferior to the PSIS. It is the attachment for the sacrotuberous ligament. Palpate by moving inferiorly from the PSIS.
Greater sciatic notch	Formed by the ilium superiorly and the ilium and ischium inferiorly. Cannot be palpated.
Greater sciatic foramen	Formed from the greater sciatic notch by ligamentous attachments. Cannot be palpated.

Ischium

Body	Makes up the entire ischium superior to the tuberosity. Cannot be palpated.
Lesser sciatic notch	Smaller cavity located on the posterior body between the greater sciatic notch and the ischial tuberosity. Cannot be palpated.
Spine	Located on the posterior body and between the greater sciatic and lesser sciatic notches. Attachment for the sacrospinous ligament. Cannot be palpated.
Tuberosity	The blunt, rough projection on the inferior part of the body. Palpate by having your partner flex at the trunk. Move your fingers up the posterior thigh to the large protuberance located slightly medial on the inferior buttock.
Ramus	Extends anteriorly from the body to connect with the inferior ramus of the pubis; is the attachment for the adductor magnus, obturator externus, and obturator internus. Palpation is usually not possible.

Pubis

Body	Main portion of the pubic bone. Palpation is difficult.
Superior ramus	Superior projection of the pubic body. Palpation is easier on self, palpate just lateral to the midline.
Inferior ramus	Inferior projection of the pubic body. It is the attachment for the inferior pubic ligament. Cannot be palpated.
Tubercle	Projects anteriorly on the superior ramus near the midline. It is the attachment for the superior pubic ligament. Not easily palpated.
Symphysis pubis	Cartilaginous joint connecting the bodies of the two pubic bones at the anterior midline. Palpation is usually not performed.

5. Ligaments function to reinforce joint capsules, and stabilize joints by influencing the movement permitted at a joint. Locate the attachments for the following ligaments on the skeleton and describe their function.

Ligament	Location	Function
Anterior sacroiliac	Attaches on the anterior surface connecting the ala and pelvic surface of the sacrum to the auricular surface of the ilium	
Interosseous sacroiliac	Attaches to the tuberosities of the ilium to the sacrum	
Short posterior sacroiliac	Attaches to the ilium and the upper portion of the sacrum on the dorsal surface	
Long posterior sacroiliac	Attaches to the posterior superior iliac spine and the lower portion of the sacrum	
Sacrotuberous	Attaches to the posterior lateral side of the sacrum inferior to the auricular surface, the coccyx, and the ischial tuberosity	
Sacrospinous	Attaches to the lower, lateral sacrum and coccyx on the posterior side and the spine of the ischium	
Iliolumbar	Attaches to the transverse process of L5 and the posterior portion of the iliac crest.	
Superior pubic	Attaches to the pubic tubercles on each side of the body	
Inferior pubic	Attaches between the inferior pubic rami	
Lumbrosacral	Attaches on the transverse process of L5 and the ala of the sacrum	

6. Using a goniometer examine the lumbrosacral angle of your partner as your partner stands in his or her normal posture and then performs anterior and posterior pelvic tilts.

   Place the axis of the goniometer at the lumbrosacral joint.

   Arrange one arm to project posteriorly and horizontal to the floor.

   Place the other arm of the goniometer vertically and parallel to the sacrum.

   Adjust the alignment of the arms as your partner moves keeping one arm horizontal and the other parallel to the sacrum.

   Note the angle formed in each position: natural, anterior tilt, and posterior tilt.

   A. Approximately what is your partner's lumbrosacral angle when in

      1) Normal posture _____

      2) Anterior tilt _____

      3) Posterior tilt _____

   B. How do the measurements you obtained compare to the normal angle of approximately 30°?

      _____

7. A. Sit in front of your standing partner. Place your thumbs on your partner's anterior superior iliac spines (ASIS).

      1) Are they level? _____ Yes _____ No
         Which is high? _____ Right _____ Left

      2) When your partner lifts the left foot off the floor without flexing the hip or knee, i.e., performs hip hiking, describe what happens to the ASISs.

         _____

      3) What happens when your partner shifts weight to the right leg and lifts the left foot off the floor by flexing the knee?

         _____

      4) Move with your partner as your partner takes one step forward with the left foot.

         What pelvic motion is produced? _____

         What motion, other than hyperextension, occurs at the right hip? _____

   B. Sit facing one side of your partner who is standing. Place one index finger on your partner's ASIS and your other index finger on your partner's posterior superior iliac spine (PSIS).

      1) Are they level? _____ Yes _____ No
         Which is high? _____ Right _____ Left

      2) What happens when your partner performs an anterior pelvic tilt?

         _____

      3) What happens when your partner performs a posterior pelvic tilt?

         _____

8. Pelvic motions are produced by force couples consisting of muscles on opposite sides of the pelvis. Examine the skeleton and perform the motions to answer the following. Circle the correct answers.

   A. Which trunk muscles when contracting concentrically produce an anterior pelvic tilt?

   Extensors   Flexors

   B. Which hip muscles would be in a position to assist the trunk muscles to produce an anterior pelvic tilt:

   Extensors   Flexors   Abductors   Adductors

   C. Which trunk muscles when contracting concentrically produce a posterior pelvic tilt?

   Extensors   Flexors

   D. Which hip muscles would be in a position to assist the trunk muscles to produce a posterior pelvic tilt:

   Extensors   Flexors   Abductors   Adductors

   E. Which trunk muscles produce a right lateral pelvic tilt?

   Left trunk flexors   Right trunk flexors

   F. Which hip muscles would be in a position to assist the trunk muscles to control a lateral pelvic tilt to the right (right side lower than left):

   Extensors   Flexors   Right abductors   Left abductors

   G. When performing a lateral pelvic tilt, the hip muscles are moving the:

   _____ Distal insertion toward the proximal insertion

   _____ Proximal insertion toward the distal insertion

■ ■ ■ Post-Lab Questions

Student's Name _____ Date Due _____

After you have completed the Worksheets and Lab Activities, answer the following questions without using your book or notes. When finished, check your answers.

1. List the pelvic motions.

   elev. / depression ,   ant. / post. Rotation   or   pro / ret. ,   anterior / post tilt

2. Describe the force couples that produce:

   A. An anterior pelvic tilt: _____ iliopsoas, Erectorspinae

   B. A posterior pelvic tilt: _____ Abs; glut Max

   C. A lateral pelvic hike: _____ Quadratus lumborum / Glut. med.

3. What motion occurs at the hip as the following are performed?

A. Anterior pelvic tilt: _____ *hip* ✓_____

B. Posterior pelvic tilt: _____ *hip* /_____

C. Pelvic rotation to the right (forward): _____ *Lt - Med. Rot. Rt - Lat, Rot.*

4. What muscle, by itself, produces hip hiking when a person is in supine?

_____ *Quadratus* _____

5. Shortness of which muscle groups will produce the following postures?

A. Anterior pelvic tilt: _____ *Abd. Ext. Erector spinae or iliopsoas* _____

B. Posterior pelvic tilt: _____ *Abd. ? Glut maximus* _____

C. In standing on the left, a lateral pelvic tilt to the right: _____ *Lt - Quadratus lumborum ↑ (Glut med.)*

6. In late stages of pregnancy, many women assume what position of the pelvis?

_____✗_____ Anterior tilt   _____ Posterior tilt   _____ Lateral tilt

Clinical Kinesiology and Anatomy of the Lower Extremities

Hip

■ ■ ■ Worksheets

Student's Name _____ Date Due _____

Complete the following questions prior to the lab class.

1. Match the following terms with their descriptors.

    A.

    ___b___ Coxa valga   A. 125°

    ___c___ Coxa varus   B. Greater than 130°

    ___A___ Angle of inclination   C. Less than 125°

    B.

    ___b___ Angle of torsion   A. Less than 15°

    ___c___ Anteversion   B. 15°–25°

    ___A___ Retroversion   C. Greater than 25°

2. On Figures 17-1, 17-2 and 17-3, label the following hip bones and landmarks. Review the landmarks of the pelvis in the previous chapters.

    B: HIP BONES: Ilium   Pubis   Ischium

    LANDMARKS: Iliac crest   ASIS   Body of pubis
                           Acetabulum   Superior ramus   PIIS
                           Inferior ramus   PSIS   Lesser sciatic notch
                           Greater sciatic notch   Ischial spine   Ischial tuberosity
                           Body of ischium   Obturator foramen   Ramus
                                                                           AIIS

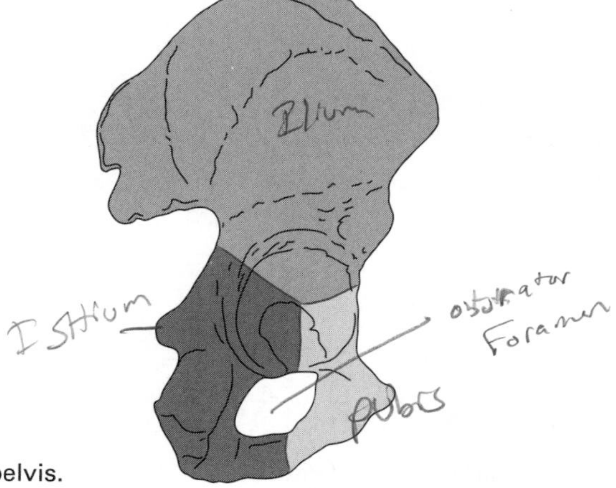

FIGURE 17-1. Landmarks of the pelvis.

FEMUR:

Head	Neck	Body
Greater trochanter	Lesser trochanter	
Medial condyle	Lateral condyle	
Medial epicondyle	Lateral epicondyle	
Linea aspera	Pectineal line	
Adductor tubercle		

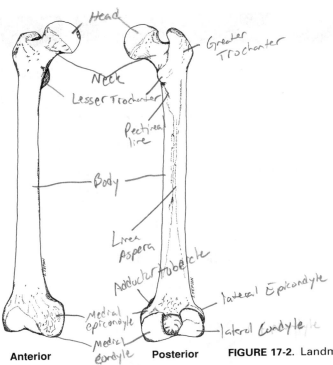

Anterior   **Posterior**   **FIGURE 17-2.** Landmarks of the femur.

TIBIA: Tibial tuberosity

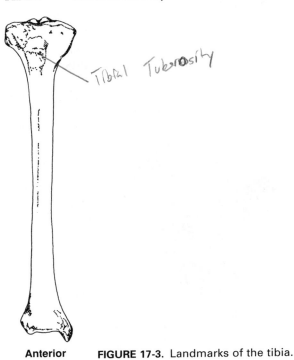

Anterior   **FIGURE 17-3.** Landmarks of the tibia.

3. On Figures 17-4 and 17-5:

   Label the following structures:

   Iliofemoral ligament   Pubofemoral ligament
   Ischiofemoral ligament

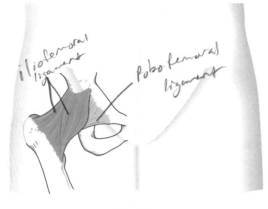 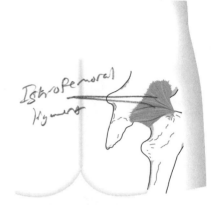

Anterior   **Posterior**

FIGURE 17-4. Ligaments of the hip.

Iliotibial band

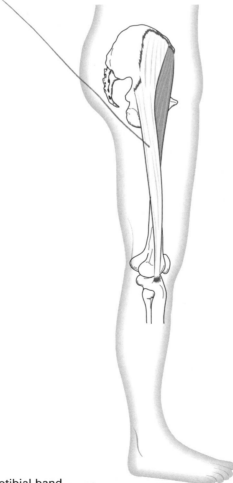

FIGURE 17-5. Iliotibial band.

4. On Figures 17-6, 17-7, 17-8, 17-9, and 17-10:

   A. Label the origin and insertion of the muscles listed.

   B. Join the origin and insertion to show the line of pull.

Iliopsoas
Pectineus

Rectus femoris
Sartorius

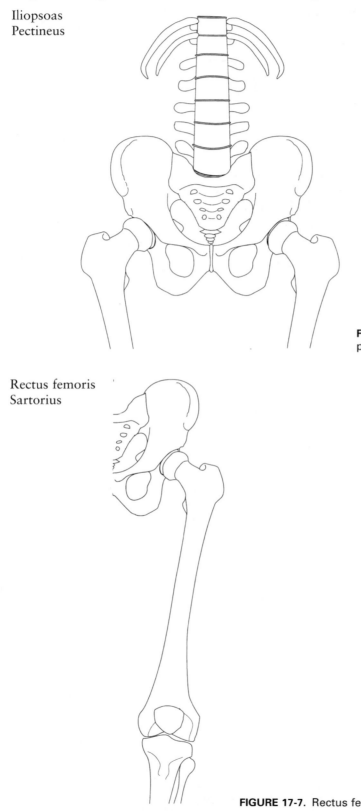

FIGURE 17-6. Iliopsoas and pectineus.

FIGURE 17-7. Rectus femoris and sartorius.

Adductor longus
Adductor brevis
Adductor magnus
Gracillis

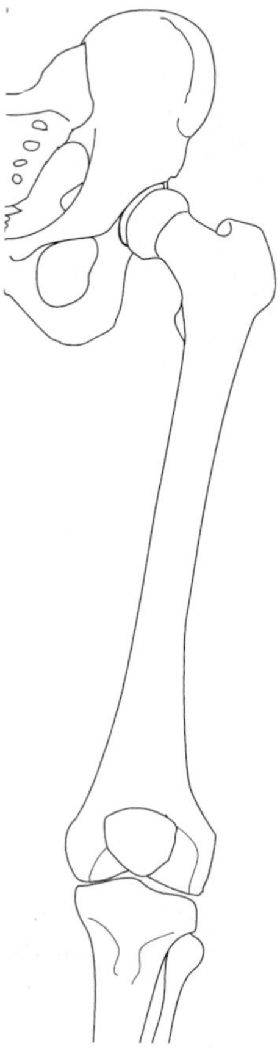

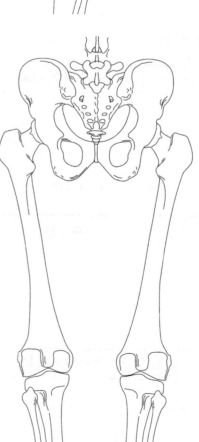

FIGURE 17-8. Adductor longus, adductor brevis, adductor magnus, and gracilis.

Gluteus maximus
Semimembranosus
Semitendinosus
Biceps femoris

FIGURE 17-9. Gluteus maximus, semimembranosus, semitendinosus, and biceps femoris.

Gluteus medius
Gluteus minimus
Tensor fascia latae

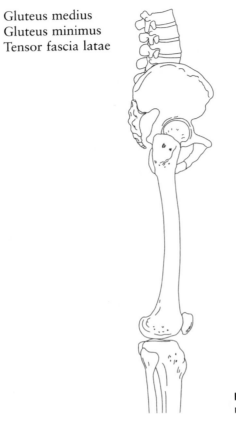

FIGURE 17-10. Gluteus medius, gluteus minimus, and tensor fascia latae.

5. For the hip joint, give the following information:

Joint	Shape	Degrees of Freedom	Motions	Plane	Axis
Hip					

6. At the hip joint, identify which surface is concave and which is convex?

Joint	Concave	Convex
Hip		

7. For the hip joint, provide the close-packed position and the loose-packed position. (Refer to Chapter 4.)

Joint	Close-Packed	Loose-Packed
Hip		

8. For the hip joint, indicate the normal end feel. (Refer to Chapter 4 for descriptions.)

   _____ Bony   _____ Capsular   _____ Soft tissue approximation

9. Match the following ligaments and structures to their function.

_____ Joint capsule	A. Reinforces hip joint capsule anteriorly
_____ Iliofemoral ligament	B. Contains blood vessels to the femoral head
_____ Pubofemoral ligament	C. Encases head and neck of femur
_____ Ischiofemoral ligament	D. Limits abduction of hip joint
_____ Ligamentum teres	E. Is insertion for gluteus maximus and tensor fascia latae
_____ Acetabular labrum	F. Assists to hold head of femur in acetabulum
_____ Inguinal ligament	G. Reinforces hip joint capsule posteriorly
_____ Iliotibial band	H. Is landmark denoting separation of trunk from the leg

10. For each hip motion listed, check the muscle(s) that are major contributors to that action.

Motion	Iliopsoas	Rectus femoris	Sartorius	Pectineus	Adductor magnus	Adductor longus	Adductor brevis	Gracilis
Flexion								
Extension								
Hyper-extension								
Abduction								
Adduction								
Medial rotation								
Lateral Rotation								

Motion	Gluteus maximus	Gluteus medius	Gluteus minimus	Semi-membranous	Semi-tendinous	Biceps femoris	Tensor fascia latae	Deep rotator group
Flexion								
Extension								
Hyper-extension								
Abduction								
Adduction								
Medial rotation								
Lateral rotation								

■ ■ ■ Lab Activities

Student's Name _____ Date Due _____

1. Perform the motions of the hip joint with your partner.
   A. Perform a motion and then your partner names the motion you performed.
   B. Your partner states a motion and then you perform that motion.

2. Using the worksheets question 5 for reference, for each of the motions available at the hip joint:
   A. Place your open left hand in the correct orientation to represent the plane of a motion.
   B. Place your right index finger to indicate the axis of that motion.
   C. Enter the plane and axis for each motion in the following chart.

Hip Joint	Plane	Axis
Flexion/extension/hyperextension		
Abduction/adduction		
Medial/lateral rotation		

3. Observe the amount of motion available at the hip joint in each plane. For each of the motions available at the hip joint, estimate the degrees of motion available by checking the box that *most closely* describes that amount of motion. (Do not measure with a goniometer.)

Motions	0°–45°	46°–90°	91°–135°	136°–180°
Flexion				
Hyperextension				
Abduction				
Adduction				
Medial rotation				
Lateral rotation				

4. Passively move your partner through the available range of motion making note of the end feel. If possible, repeat with several people. Review question 8 in the worksheets for the normal end feel.

   A. Is your partner's end feel consistent with what the end feel is reported to be?

   _____

   B. What structures create the end feel for this joint?

   _____

   _____

5. On the skeleton, anatomical models, and at least one partner, locate, palpate, and observe the following structures. The reference position is the anatomical position. Having pictures for reference is helpful when trying to find structures. Not all structures are palpable on your partner. Review Chapter 16 "Pelvic Girdle" for structures on the ischium and pubis.

Ilium

Iliac fossa	Large, smooth, concave area on the internal surface; attachment for the iliopsoas muscle. It cannot be palpated because of the iliopsoas muscle and abdominal contents. From just above the ASIS on the iliac crest, however, you may be able to roll your fingers over into the fossa area.

(Continued...)

Ilium *(continued)*

Iliac crest	Superior margin of ilium extending from the ASIS to the PSIS. Iliac crests appear to be located more superiorly in men than women. Palpate by placing your hand on the top margin of the pelvis. 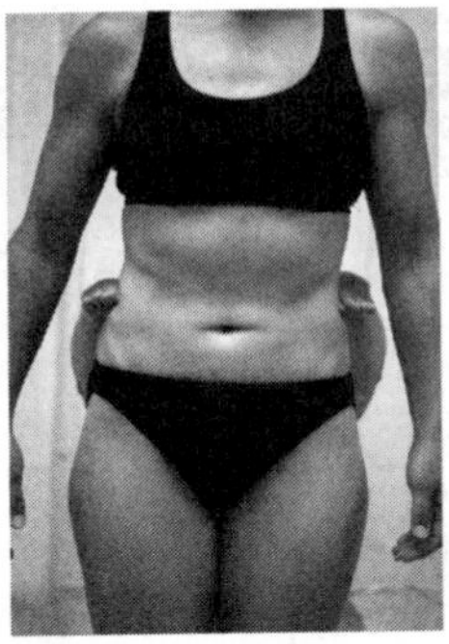 **FIGURE 17-11.** Palpating the iliac crest.
Anterior superior iliac spine (ASIS)	The projection on the anterior end of the iliac crest; attachment for the tensor fascia latae, sartorius, and inguinal ligament. Palpate by move to the anterior most point of the iliac crest. 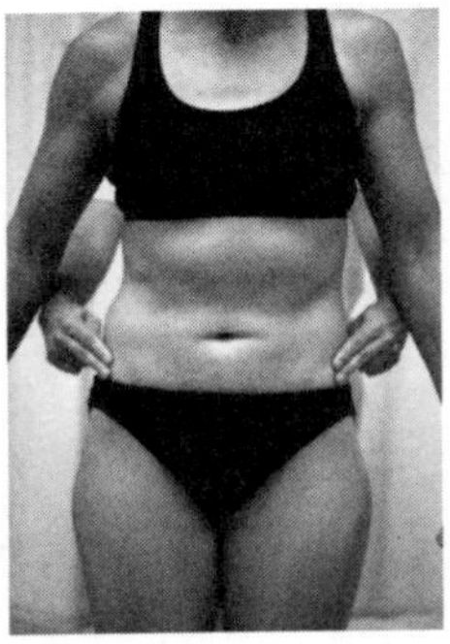 **FIGURE 17-12.** Palpating the ASIS.
Anterior inferior iliac spine (AIIS)	The projection just inferior to the ASIS; attachment for the rectus femoris. Can be difficult to palpate as it is deep to muscle.
Posterior superior iliac spine (PSIS)	Posterior projection of the iliac crest. It is the attachment for the posterior sacroiliac ligaments. Palpate by placing your hand on the iliac crest and moving posterior and medially to the first protuberance. A "dimple" is usually observable over the PSIS. 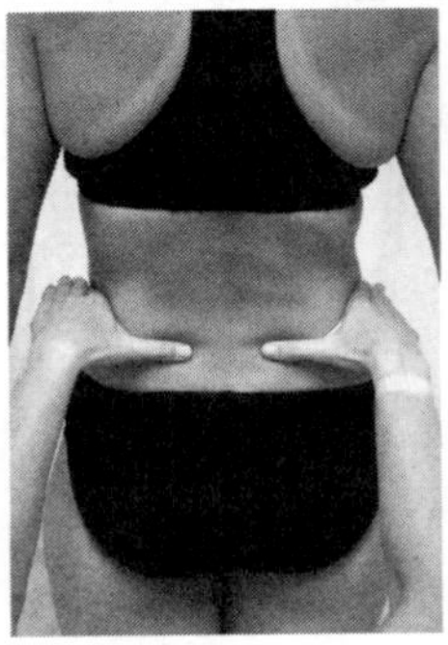 **FIGURE 17-13.** Palpating the PSIS.
Posterior inferior iliac spine (PIIS)	Protuberance located inferior to the PSIS. It is the attachment for the sacrotuberous ligament. Palpate by moving inferiorly from the PSIS.

Femur

Head	Rounded portion on the proximal medial border of the femur; articulates with the acetabulum. Cannot be palpated.
Neck	Narrow portion located between the head and the trochanters. Cannot be palpated.
Greater trochanter	Large protuberance located on the proximal lateral aspect between the neck and the body of the femur. It is the attachment for the gluteus medius and minimus, and most deep rotators. Easily palpated by placing your fingers on the proximal lateral aspect of the femur and then as the femur is rotated the greater trochanter can be felt as it rolls under your fingers. 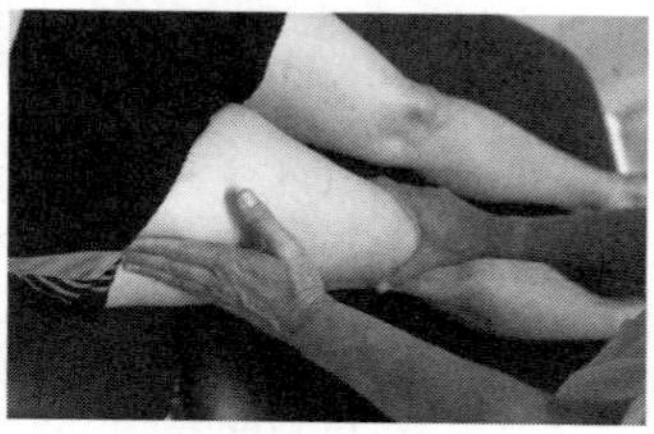 **FIGURE 17-14.** Palpating the greater trochanter.
Lesser trochanter	Smaller protuberance located slightly posteriorly on the proximal, medial femur distal to the greater trochanter; attachment for the iliopsoas. Palpation is usually not possible.
Shaft or body	Long cylindrical portion, bowed slightly anteriorly; attachment for the hamstrings and quadriceps. Palpation is usually not possible.
Medial condyle	Rounded portion on the distal medial end just proximal to the knee joint. With the knee flexed and muscles relaxed, palpate on the medial side. 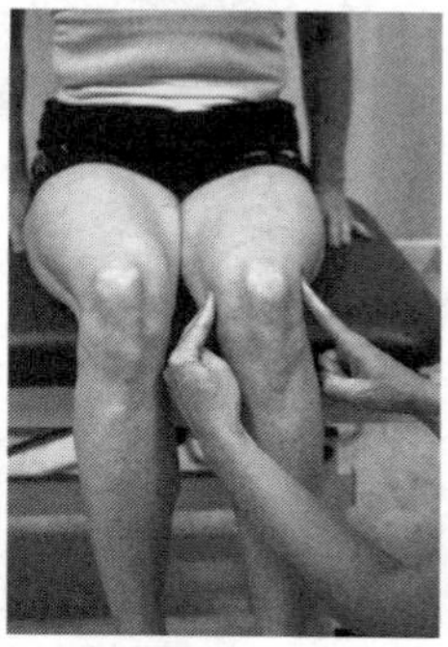 **FIGURE 17-15.** Palpating the medial and lateral condyles. Left index finger showing medial condyle. Right index finger showing lateral condyle.
Lateral condyle	Rounded portion on the distal lateral end just proximal to the knee joint. With the knee flexed and the muscle relaxed, palpate on the lateral side. See Figure 17-15.
Medial epicondyle	Projection proximal to the medial condyle. With the knee flexed, move your fingers medially to the inside of the knee and proximal to the medial condyle.
Lateral epicondyle	Projection proximal to the lateral condyle. With the knee flexed, move your fingers laterally to the outside of the knee and proximal to the lateral condyle.

(Continued...)

Femur *(continued)*

Adductor tubercle	Small projection proximal to the medial epicondyle. It is the attachment for a portion of the adductor magnus. With the knee extended, find the spot just superior to the medial epicondyle. Move your fingers back and forth across the adductor magnus tendon. Usually tender to touch.
Linea aspera	Prominent longitudinal ridge or crest running most of the length of the posterior side. Cannot be palpated.
Patellar surface	Located on the distal anterior surface between the condyles. Articulates with the posterior surface of the patella. The patellar surface can be palpated when the knee is fully flexed and the patella has moved distally. Place your fingers just above the superior border of the patella. Do not move your fingers as you flex the knee.

Tibia

Tibial tuberosity	Large projection located on the proximal anterior midline of the tibia; attachment for the patellar tendon. Often visually evident, palpation is easy. With the knee flexed and the muscle relaxed, palpate by moving distally from the patella along the patellar tendon to the insertion (Fig. 17-16). 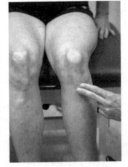 **FIGURE 17-16.** Palpating the tibial tuberosity.

Ligaments and Other Structures

Iliofemoral ligament or "Y" ligament	Crosses the joint anteriorly from the AIIS to the intertrochanteric line of the femur—a line between the greater and lesser trochanters. Because the ligament splits before inserting on the femur, it resembles the letter "Y." Cannot be palpated.
Pubofemoral ligament	Crosses the hip on the medial inferior side passing posteriorly and inferiorly from the medial aspect of the acetabular rim and superior ramus of the pubis to the neck of the femur. Cannot be palpated.
Ischiofemoral ligament	Crosses the hip on the posterior side passing laterally and proximally from the ischial portion of the acetabulum to the femoral neck. Cannot be palpated.
Ligamentum teres	A small intercapsular ligament that attaches to the acetabulum and the fovea of the femoral head. Cannot be palpated.

(Continued...)

Acetabular labrum	Located around the rim of the acetabulum thereby increasing the depth of the acetabulum and surrounding the head of the femur, contributes to holding the head in the acetabulum. Cannot be palpated.
Inguinal ligament	Located on the anterior surface, it serves as the boundary between the trunk and the lower extremity. With the knees and hips slightly flexed and relaxed (support on a bolster), palpate the ASIS and then move your fingers diagonally downward to the symphysis pubis (in the bend of the hip). Move your fingers back and forth across the ligament. Just distal to this, palpate the femoral pulse as the femoral artery and vein pass under it.
Iliotibial band or tract (IT band)	Located on the lateral aspect of the thigh attaching to the anterior portion of the iliac crest and the proximal anterior lateral tibia. Attachment for the gluteus maximus and tensor fascia latae. Palpate the tendon of the biceps femoris located posterior and proximal to the knee. Palpate the IT band lateral to the biceps femoris tendon. Move your fingers side to side across the IT band. Extending and adducting the hip may cause the IT band to be more prominent on the lateral side of the thigh.

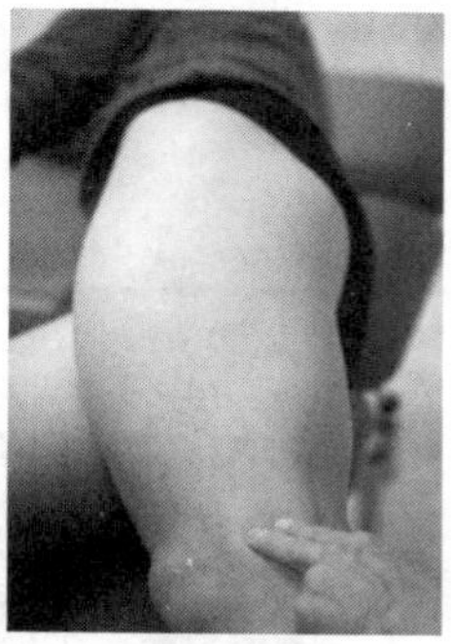

FIGURE 17-17. Palpating the IT band.

6. Use a disarticulated skeleton or anatomical model of the hip joint and apply the rules of joint arthrokinematics and the concave-convex rule to perform the following exercises.

A. Underline the correct answer.

The acetabulum is: Concave   Convex

The femur is: Concave   Convex

B. Move the femur in the acetabulum in all planes of motion.

C. Observe the movement of the femur on the acetabulum. Circle the motions that you observed.

Roll   Spin   Glide

D. Observe the movement of the distal end of the femur in relation to the movement of the proximal end of the femur as you move the femur in the acetabulum. Does the

distal end of the femur move in the _____ same or _____ opposite direction as the proximal end of the femur?

7. Locate the following on the skeleton, anatomical models, and at least one partner:

A. Locate the origin and insertion of the muscle on the skeleton.

B. Stretch a large rubber band taut by placing one end at the origin and the other end at the insertion of a muscle on the skeleton.

C. Perform the motion that the muscle does and observe how the rubber band becomes less taut and shorter, similar to the muscle shortening as it contracts.

D. Perform the opposite motion and observe how the rubber band becomes tauter and longer, similar to the muscle lengthening as it is being stretched.

E. After locating the muscle on the skeleton, locate the muscle on your partner. The position described for locating the muscle on your partner is the manual muscle test position for a fair or better grade of muscle strength. Not all origins, insertions, and muscle bellies can be palpated on your partner.

F. When possible, palpate the origin, insertion, and muscle belly of each muscle by:

1) Placing your fingers on the origin and insertion, and asking your partner to contract the muscle.

2) Moving your fingers from the origin and insertion over the contracting muscle.

3) Asking your partner to relax the muscle and again moving your fingers from the origin to the insertion over the muscle.

4) Note the difference between the contracting and relaxed muscles.

G. In the following tables, information needed to palpate each muscle is provided. The information includes position of the person, origin and insertion of the muscle, the line of pull of the muscle, the muscle's action, instructions to give to the person to make the muscle contract, and, finally, information on the best location to palpate the muscle.

Sitting Position

ILIOPSOAS	A deep muscle located on the anterior aspect of the hip joint.
FIGURE 17-18. Palpating the iliopsoas.
Position of person:	Sitting with hip and knee in about 90° of flexion and neutral alignment.
Origin:	Anterior surface of the iliac fossa, the anterior and lateral surfaces of the vertebral bodies and the transverse processes of T12–L5.
Insertion:	Lesser trochanter of the femur.
Line of pull:	Vertical on the anterior surface of the hip joint.
Muscle action:	Hip flexion.
Palpate:	At the midline in the "bend" of the hip, distal to the inguinal ligament.
Instructions to person:	Flex your hip, lift your thigh straight up and off the table.

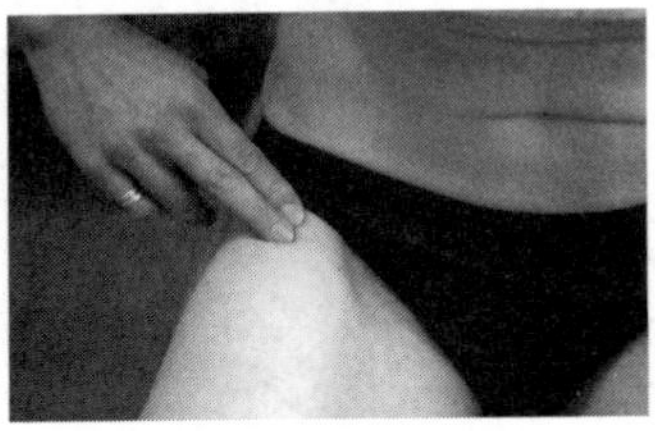

(Continued...)

RECTUS FEMORIS	A superficial muscle located on the anterior thigh. This muscle is one part of the quadriceps muscle.
	FIGURE 17-19. Palpating the rectus femoris.
Position of person:	Sitting with hip and knee in about 90° of flexion and neutral alignment.
Origin:	Anterior inferior iliac spine.
Insertion:	Tibial tuberosity via the patellar tendon.
Line of pull:	Vertical on the anterior surface of the hip joint.
Muscle action:	Hip flexion and knee extension.
Palpate:	As it crosses anterior to the hip joint lateral to the iliopsoas.
Instructions to person:	Flex your hip, lift your thigh straight up and off the table.
SARTORIUS	A superficial muscle located anterior to the hip joint and medially on the thigh.
	FIGURE 17-20. Palpating the sartorius.
Position of person:	Sitting with hip and knee in about 90° of flexion and neutral alignment.
Origin:	Anterior superior iliac spine.
Insertion:	Proximal medial tibia.
Line of pull:	Diagonal on the anterior surface of the hip joint.
Muscle action:	Simultaneous hip flex, abduction, and lateral rotation and knee flexion.
Palpate:	Near the origin or as it crosses diagonally across the thigh.
Instructions to person:	Flex your hip, lift your thigh off the table as you place your ankle on the opposite knee.

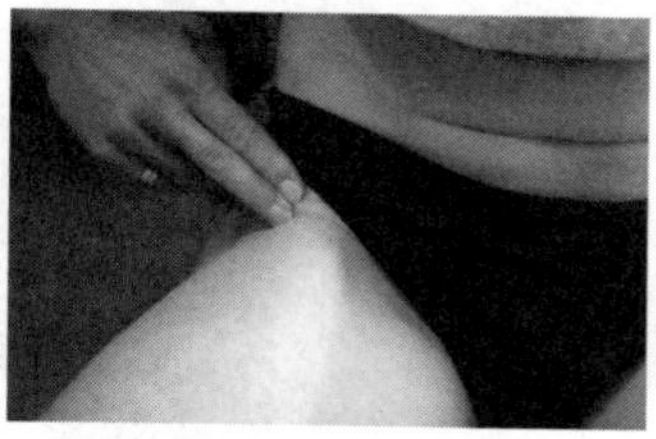

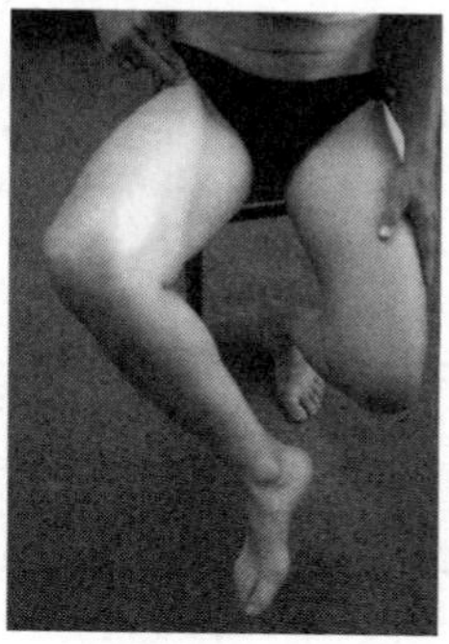

Side-lying Position on Same Side as Muscle Being Examined

PECTINEUS	Located medially and inferior to the hip joint between the adductor longus medially and the iliopsoas laterally. **FIGURE 17-21.** Palpating pectineus.
Position of person:	Hip and knee on side being examined in midline, opposite hip and knee flexed with foot on supporting surface or supported in abduction by the examiner.
Origin:	Superior ramus of the pubis.
Insertion:	Pectineal line of the femur.
Line of pull:	Diagonal.
Muscle action:	Hip flexion and adduction. The hip lifting the leg off the supporting surface maintains neutral alignment.
Palpate:	Palpate on the proximal medial aspect of the thigh.
Instructions to person:	Lift your leg up toward the ceiling.
GRACILIS	A superficial muscle located on the medial thigh.
Position of person:	Hip and knee on side being examined in midline, opposite hip and knee flexed with foot on supporting surface.
Origin:	Pubis.
Insertion:	Proximal anterior medial tibia.
Line of pull:	Vertical on the medial surface of the hip joint.
Muscle action:	Hip adduction.
Palpate:	Palpate on the medial thigh. The adductors are relatively close together and all perform similar motions. Distinguishing between the muscles can be difficult.
Instructions to person:	Lift your leg up toward the ceiling.
ADDUCTOR MAGNUS	Located on the medial thigh deep to the adductor longus, brevis, and gracilis muscles and anterior to the medial hamstrings.
Position of person:	Hip and knee on side being examined in midline, opposite hip and knee flexed with foot on supporting surface.
Origin:	Ischial tuberosity and pubis.
Insertion:	Entire linea aspera and adductor tubercle.

(Continued...)

Line of pull:	Diagonal on the medial surface of the hip joint.
Muscle action:	Hip adduction.
Palpate:	Locate the ischial tuberosity, move slightly forward on the medial aspect of the thigh. Another place to palpate is the distal attachment at the adductor tubercle.
Instructions to person:	Lift your leg up toward the ceiling.
ADDUCTOR LONGUS	A superficial muscle on the medial thigh.
Position of person:	Hip and knee on side being examined in midline, opposite hip and knee flexed with foot on supporting surface.
Origin:	Pubis.
Insertion:	Middle third of the linea aspera of the femur.
Line of pull:	Diagonal on the medial surface of the hip joint.
Muscle action:	Hip adduction.
Palpate:	Palpate on the proximal medial thigh. The adductors are relatively close together and all perform the same motion. Distinguishing between the muscles can be difficult.
Instructions to person:	Lift your leg toward the ceiling.
ADDUCTOR BREVIS	Located deep to the adductor longus muscle.
Position of person:	Hip and knee on side being examined in midline, opposite hip and knee flexed with foot on supporting surface.
Origin:	Pubis.
Insertion:	Pectineal line and proximal linea aspera of the femur.
Line of pull:	Diagonal on the medial surface of the hip joint.
Muscle action:	Hip adduction.
Palpate:	Palpate on the proximal medial thigh. The adductors are relatively close together and all perform the same motion. Distinguishing between the muscles can be difficult.
Instructions to person:	Lift your leg toward the ceiling.

Prone Position

GLUTEUS MAXIMUS	A superficial muscle on the posterior pelvis.

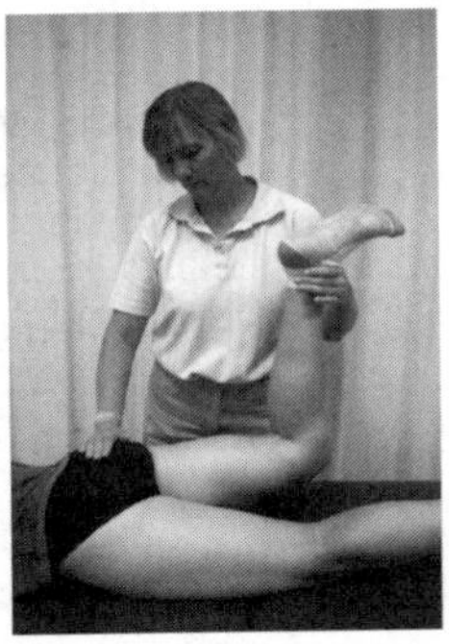

FIGURE 17-22. Palpating the gluteus maximus.

Position of person:	Hip in neutral alignment, knee flexed to about 90°.
Origin:	Posterior surfaces of the sacrum and ilium.
Insertion:	Posterior femur distal to the greater trochanter and iliotibial band.
Line of pull:	Diagonal on the posterior surface of the hip joint.
Muscle action:	Hip extension, hyperextension, and lateral rotation. Extend the hip, lift the thigh off the supporting surface maintaining neutral alignment.
Palpate:	Over the center of the buttocks.
Instructions to person:	Lift your leg off the table keeping your knee bent.

SEMITENDINOSUS	A superficial muscle on the posterior medial aspect of the thigh.

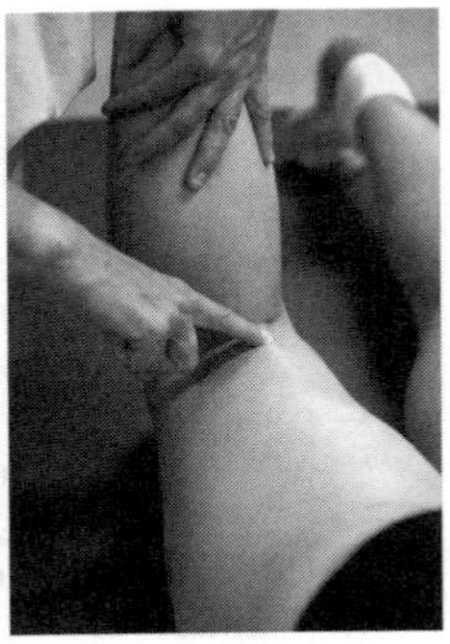

FIGURE 17-23. Palpating the semitendinosus.

Position of person:	Hip and knee extended and in neutral alignment.
Origin:	Ischial tuberosity.
Insertion:	Proximal anterior medial tibia.
Line of pull:	Vertical on the posterior surface of the hip joint.
Muscle action:	Hip extension and knee flexion.

(Continued...)

Prone Position *(continued)*

Palpate:	Palpate on the posterior medial thigh. The long distal tendon is on the distal medial aspect of the thigh superficial to the attachment of the semimembranosus.
Instructions to person:	Lift your leg off the table keeping your knee bent.
SEMIMEMBRANOSUS	Deep to the semitendinosus muscle and located on the posterior medial thigh (Fig. 17-24). 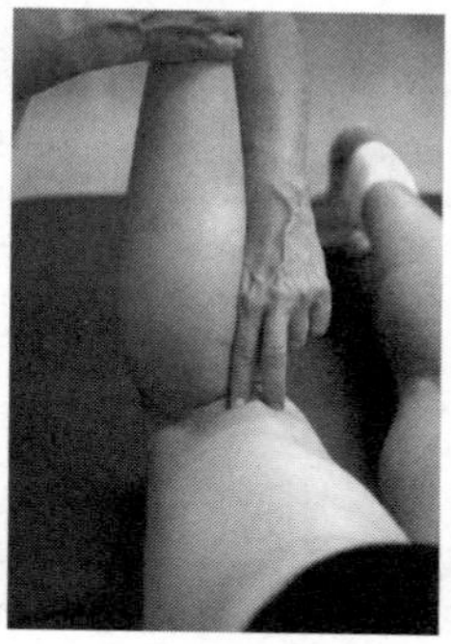 **FIGURE 17-24.** Palpating the semimembranosus.
Position of person:	Hip and knee extended and in neutral alignment.
Origin:	Ischial tuberosity.
Insertion:	Posterior surface of the medial condyle of the tibia.
Line of pull:	Vertical on the posterior surface of the hip joint.
Muscle action:	Hip extension and knee flexion.
Palpate:	Palpate on the posterior medial thigh. Distinguishing between the semimembranosus and the semitendinosus can be difficult. The semimembranosus has a broad attachment on the posterior surface of the tibia deep to, and on either side of, the semitendinosus just above the knee joint.
Instructions to person:	Lift your leg off the table keeping your knee bent.
BICEPS FEMORIS	A superficial muscle on the posterior lateral thigh. 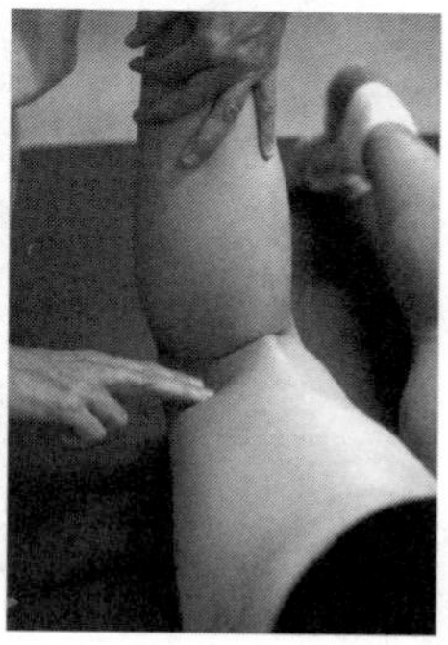 **FIGURE 17-25.** Palpating the biceps femoris.
Position of person:	Hip and knee extended and in neutral alignment.
Origin:	Long head: Ischial tuberosity. Short head: Lateral lip of the linea aspera of the femur.

(Continued...)

Prone Position *(continued)*

Insertion:	Posterior proximal fibular head.
Line of pull:	Vertical on the posterior surface of the hip joint.
Muscle action:	Long head: Hip extension and knee flexion. Short head: Knee flexion.
Palpate:	Palpate on the posterior lateral thigh. The tendon is palpated on the distal lateral thigh at the knee joint.
Instructions to person:	Lift your leg off the table keeping your knee bent.
DEEP ROTATORS	Deep muscles. Hip rotation is usually examined in sitting, however, to palpate the muscles the person is in prone.
Position of person:	Hip in extension and neutral rotation and knee in about 90° of flexion.
Origin:	Posterior sacrum, ischium, and pubis.
Insertion:	Areas of the greater trochanter.
Line of pull:	Horizontal on the posterior surface of the hip joint.
Muscle action:	Hip lateral rotation.
Palpate:	Palpation is generally difficult except the piriformis. With one hand locate the PSIS. With the other hand, locate the coccyx. These landmarks form a "T," with the piriformis located along the base of the "T." Press on the muscle and have your partner laterally rotate the hip. You may be able to feel the piriformis contracting under the gluteus maximus.
Instructions to person:	Keeping your thigh on the table, roll your leg out (heel in, toe out).

Side-lying on Side Opposite Muscle Being Examined

GLUTEUS MEDIUS	Mostly deep to the gluteus maximus on the posterior and lateral pelvis, except the upper fibers, which are superficial. **FIGURE 17-26.** Palpating the gluteus medius.
Position of person:	Hip and knee extended in neutral alignment and the lower leg slightly flexed at hip and knee for greater stability.
Origin:	Outer surface of the ilium.

(Continued...)

Insertion:	Lateral surface of the greater trochanter of the femur.
Line of pull:	Vertical on the lateral surface of the hip joint.
Muscle action:	Abduction.
Palpate:	Palpate on the proximal lateral pelvis and at the insertion on the greater trochanter. Also palpate in the area just below the iliac crest between the PSIS and the ASIS. May be difficult to distinguish from the gluteus minimus.
Instructions to person:	Lift your top leg to the ceiling.
GLUTEUS MINIMUS	On the lateral pelvis deep to the gluteus medius 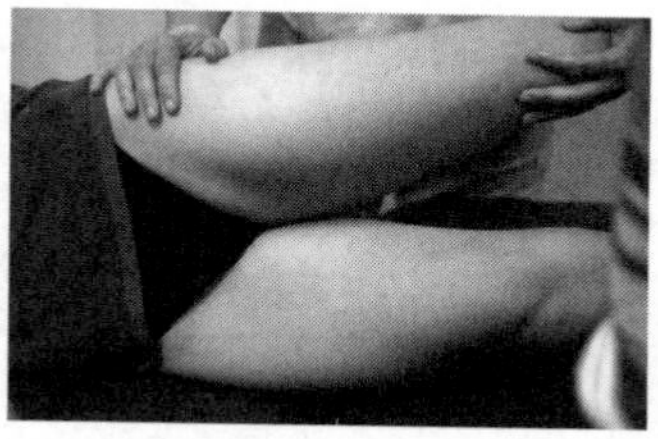 . FIGURE 17-27. Palpating the gluteus minimus.
Position of person:	Hip and knee extended in neutral alignment and the lower leg slightly flexed at hip and knee for greater stability.
Origin:	Outer surface of the ilium.
Insertion:	Anterior surface of the greater trochanter.
Line of pull:	Diagonal on the lateral surface of the hip joint.
Muscle action:	Hip abduction, medial rotation.
Palpate:	Palpate on the lateral aspect of the pelvis and at the insertion. Difficult to distinguish form the gluteus medius.
Instructions to person:	Lift your top leg to the ceiling.
TENSOR FASCIA LATAE	A superficial muscle on the proximal anterior lateral thigh between the rectus femoris and the gluteus medius. 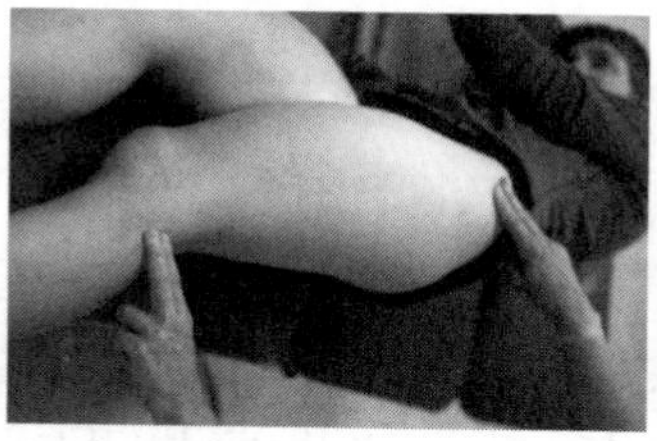 FIGURE 17-28. Palpating near the origin and insertion of the tensor fascia latae.
Position of person:	Hip and knee extended in neutral alignment and the lower leg slightly flexed at hip and knee for greater stability.
Origin:	Anterior superior iliac spine.

(Continued...)

Side-lying on Side Opposite Muscle Being Examined *(continued)*

Insertion:	Lateral condyle of the tibia via the iliotibial band.
Line of pull:	Diagonal on the lateral surface of the hip joint.
Muscle action:	Combined hip flexion and abduction.
Palpate:	Palpate the muscle on the proximal anterior lateral thigh slightly distal and posterior from the ASIS and the iliotibial band on the lateral thigh.
Instructions to person:	Lift your top leg toward the ceiling.

8. For the multijoint muscles of the hip, indicate the positions that simultaneous lengthen or shorten them over all the joints they cross.

Muscle	Lengthened Position		Shortened Position	
	Hip	Knee	Hip	Knee
Sartorius				
Semitendinosus				
Semimembranosus				
Biceps femoris—long head				
Rectus femoris				
Gracilis				
Tensor fascia latae				

9. A person's manual muscle test grade of the left gluteus maximus is 3+ (fair plus), which means the person can move through full range of motion against gravity. (Review Chapter 5 for muscle strength grades.) What position of the knee should the person maintain while performing strengthening exercises of the gluteus maximus muscle? Why?

_____

_____

10. After being hit on the R lateral pelvis by another player's helmet in a football game 2 weeks ago, the middle line backer is experiencing weakness of his right hip abductors. You are to design a strengthening program for him. Diagram the lever that describes hip abduction performed in the supine position.

   A. Draw a stick figure performing right hip abduction in supine.

   B. Draw an arrow to indicate the direction of the movement.

C. Draw a line to indicate the hip abductor muscles.

11. Analyze the activity of hip abduction diagrammed in question 10 by answering the following questions:

A. Which joint motion is being analyzed? _____

B. Identify the "axis" of the motion: _____

C. Would gravity cause the movement? _____

D. Is the "resistance" to the movement a muscle or the weight of the leg? _____

E. Which major muscle group is the agonist? _____

F. Which major muscle group is the antagonist? _____

G. Is the agonist performing a concentric or an eccentric contraction? _____

H. Is the antagonist active? _____

I. Is this an open or closed kinetic chain activity? _____

12. The middle line backer has improved the strength of his right hip abductors and has progressed to performing hip abductor strengthening exercises in side-lying on the left. Diagram the lever that describes hip abduction performed in the side-lying position. Analyze the motion of lifting the leg toward the ceiling.

A. Draw a stick figure performing hip abduction in side-lying.

B. Draw arrows to indicate the direction of the movement, the direction of the pull of the muscle, and the direction of gravity.

C. Label the arrow that represents force with an "F" and the arrow that represents resistance with an "R."

13. Analyze the activity of hip abduction diagrammed in question 12 by answering the following questions:

   A. Which joint motion is being analyzed? _____

   B. Identify the "axis" of the motion: _____

   C. Would gravity cause the movement? _____

   D. Is the muscle acting to overcome gravity or slow down gravity? _____

   E. Is the "resistance" to the movement a muscle or gravity? _____

   F. Which major muscle group is the agonist? _____

   G. Which major muscle group is the antagonist? _____

   H. Is the agonist performing a concentric or an eccentric contraction? _____

   I. Is the antagonist active? _____

   J. Is this an open or closed kinetic chain activity? _____

14. The middle line backer is still performing hip abduction in side-lying. This time, analyze the motion of lowering the leg to the supporting surface. Diagram the lever that describes lowering the hip from the abducted position.

   A. Draw a stick figure performing hip adduction in side-lying.

   B. Draw arrows to indicate the direction of the movement, the direction of the pull of the muscle, and the direction of gravity.

   C. Label the arrow that represents force with an "F" and the arrow that represents resistance with an "R."

15. Analyze the activity of hip adduction diagrammed in question 14 by answering the following questions:

   A. Which joint motion is being analyzed? _____

   B. Identify the "axis" of the motion: _____

   C. Would gravity cause the movement? _____

   D. Is the muscle acting to overcome gravity or slow down gravity? _____

   E. Is the "resistance" to the movement a muscle or gravity? _____

   F. Which major muscle group is the agonist? _____

   G. Which major muscle group is the antagonist? _____

   H. Is the agonist performing a concentric or an eccentric contraction? _____

I. Is the antagonist active? _____

J. Is this an open or closed kinetic chain activity? _____

16. The middle line backer wants to return to play. You have one more exercise you want him to do. He is to perform right hip abductor strengthening exercises standing on his right leg while flexing his left hip and knee. Diagram the lever that describes the action at the right hip when standing on the right leg only.

A. Draw a stick figure performing standing on the right leg and lifting the left leg off the floor.

B. Indicate the location of the right hip abductors.

C. Indicate what the resistance is.

17. Analyze the activity of hip abduction diagrammed in question 16 by answering the following questions:

A. Which joint motion is being analyzed? _____

B. Identify the "axis" of the motion: _____

C. Would gravity cause the movement? _____

D. Is the muscle acting to overcome gravity or slow down gravity? _____

E. Is the "resistance" to the movement a muscle or gravity? _____

F. Which major muscle group is the agonist? _____

G. Which major muscle group is the antagonist? _____

H. What type of contraction is the agonist performing? _____

I. Is the antagonist active? _____

J. Is this an open or closed kinetic chain activity? _____

■ ■ ■ Post-Lab Questions

Student's Name _____ Date Due _____

After you have completed the Worksheets and Lab Activities, answer the following questions without using your book or notes. When finished, check your answers.

1. A. List the combined joint motions required to put your right ankle on your left knee when you are in a sitting position.

   _____

   B. What muscle performs the motions described in A above?

   _____

2. Name the hip muscle that has an attachment on the lumbar spine.

   _____

3. List, in order starting from the anterior midline and proceeding laterally around the knee, the hip muscles that attach below the knee.

   _____

   _____

4. Generally, the following muscle groups share innervation from which peripheral nerves:

   Hamstrings: _____

   Hip flexors: _____

   Hip adductors: _____

5. Applying a deep heat treatment to the posterior lateral pelvis heats the muscles in the area. List the muscles in the order in which they will be heated if the heat penetrates from the most superficial to the deepest muscle.

   _____

   _____

6. The acetabulum is located on the _____ surface of the hip joint.

7. You are to design an exercise program for a person with a problem with her hip. To design the exercise program, you need to know the muscles that attached to the:

   A. Ischial tuberosity. List the muscles that attach to the ischial tuberosity.

   _____

   B. ASIS and AIIS. List the muscles that attach to the ASIS and AIIS.

   ASIS

   _____

   AIIS

   _____

8. Of the deep rotators of the hip, the piriformis is clinically significant as it can cause nerve compression. Which nerve is in a position to be compressed by the piriformis muscle?

_____

9. You are assisting family members to learn to position their thin, frail father who has advanced Parkinson's disease. What bony landmarks must you educate them about for each of the following positions?

Prone:

_____

Supine:

_____

Side-lying:

_____

Knee

■ ■ ■ Worksheets

Student's Name _____ Date Due _____

Complete the following questions prior to the lab class.

1. Define Q angle: _____
   _____

2. List the muscles that make up the pes anserine. _____
   _____

3. Match the following terms descriptive of alignment of the lower extremity with the
   appropriate description.

   _____ Genu valgum   A. Knee joint in more than 0° of extension

   _____ Genu varum   B. Ankle more lateral than normal

   _____ Genu recurvatum   C. Ankle more medial than normal

4. On Figures 18-1 and 18-2, label the following bones, landmarks, and joints:

   TIBIA: Intercondylar eminence   Medial condyle
               Lateral condyle   Tibial plateau
               Tibial tuberosity   Medial malleolus
               Crest

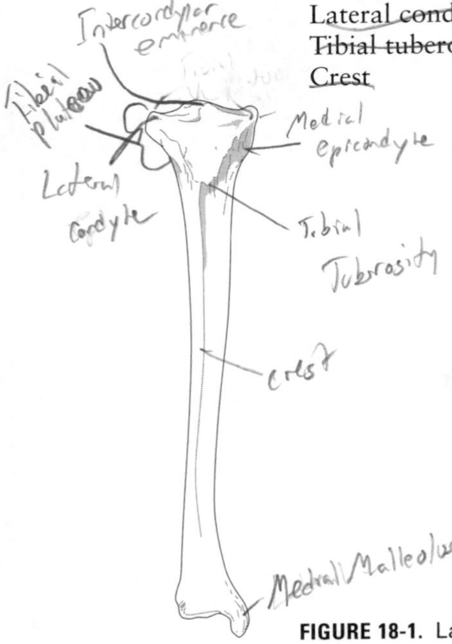

FIGURE 18-1. Landmarks of the tibia.

BONES: Fibula   Tibia   Patella   Calcaneus

JOINTS: Patellofemoral   Knee

LANDMARKS: Fibular head   Lateral malleolus
                    Patellar articular surface

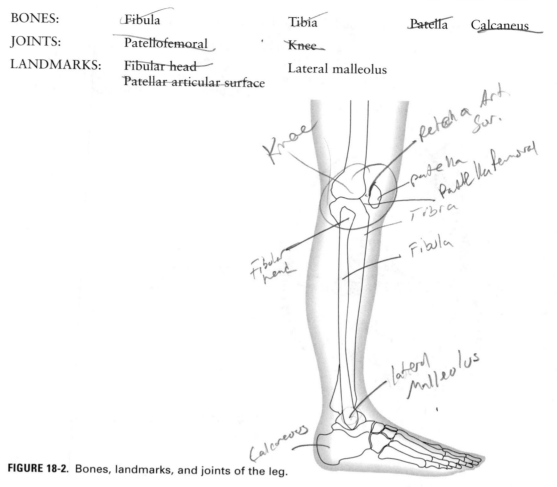

FIGURE 18-2. Bones, landmarks, and joints of the leg.

5. On Figures 18-3 A & B:

   Label the following structures of the knee:

   A. Anterior cruciate   Posterior cruciate

   B. The three parts of the pes anserine

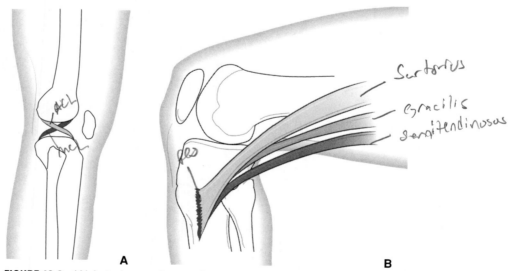

FIGURE 18-3. *(A)* Anterior cruciate and posterior cruciate. *(B)* Pes anserine.

C. On Figure18-4, label the following structures of the knee:

Medial collateral ligament   Lateral collateral ligament   Medial meniscus
Lateral meniscus   Lateral tibial condyle   Lateral femoral condyle
Medial tibial condyle   Medial femoral condyle   Tibial tuberosity
Fibular head   Transverse Ligament   Posterior cruciate ligament
Anterior cruciate ligament

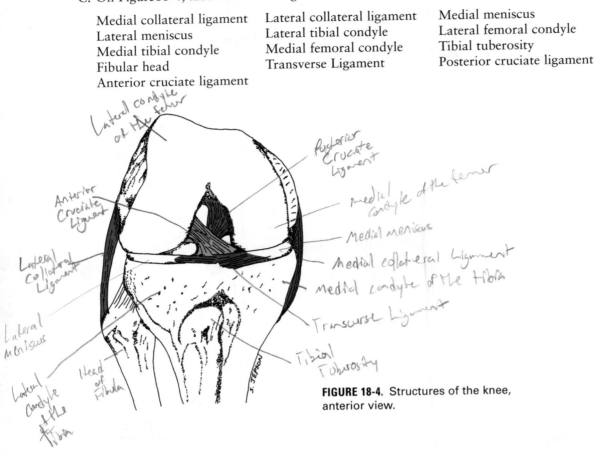

FIGURE 18-4. Structures of the knee, anterior view.

6. On Figures 18-5 and 18-6:

A. Label the origin and insertion of the muscles listed.

B. Join the origin and insertion to show the line of pull.

C. Review semimembranosus, semitendinosus, and biceps femoris in Chapter 17.

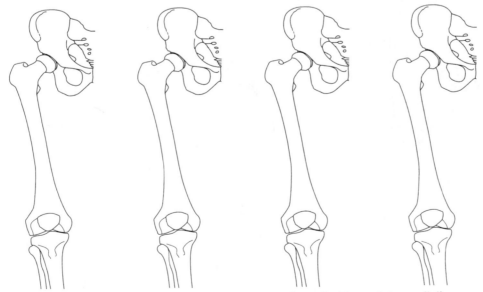

FIGURE 18-5. Rectus femoris. Vastus medialis. Vastus lateralis. Vastus intermedialis.

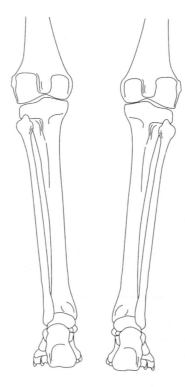

FIGURE 18-6. Popliteus and gastrocnemius.

7. For the knee joint, give the following information:

Joint	Shape	Degrees of Freedom	Motions	Plane	Axis
Knee					

8. At the knee joint, identify which surface is concave and which is convex.

Joint	Concave	Convex
Knee		

9. For the knee joint, provide the close-packed position and the loose-packed position. (Refer to Chapter 4.)

Joint	Close-Packed	Loose-Packed
Knee		

10. For the knee joint, describe the normal end feel. (Refer to Chapter 4 for descriptions.)

   Flexion: _____ Bony   _____ Capsular   _____ Soft tissue approximation

   Extension: _____ Bony   _____ Capsular   _____ Soft tissue approximation

11. Match each ligament and structure that follows with the appropriate function or characteristic. An answer may be used more than once. Each function or characteristic may have more than one correct answer.

    A. Provides stability in the frontal plane.

    B. Prevents anterior displacement of the tibia on the femur.

    C. Fibers of the meniscus attach to this ligament.

    D. Deepens the joint surface.

    E. Prevents posterior displacement of the tibia on the femur.

    F. Absorbs shock.

    _____ Posterior cruciate ligament

    _____ Anterior cruciate ligament

    _____ Lateral collateral ligament

    _____ Medial collateral ligament

    _____ Lateral meniscus

    _____ Medial meniscus

12. For each muscle listed, check the motions for which the muscle is a major contributor at the knee.

Muscle	Flexion	Extension
Vastus lateralis		
Vastus medialis		
Vastus intermedialis		
Rectus femoris		
Semimembranosus		
Semitendinosus		
Biceps femoris		
Popliteus		
Gastrocnemius		

13. For the multijoint muscles, indicate the positions that simultaneously lengthen or shorten them over all the joints they cross.

Muscle	Lengthened Position			Shortened Position		
	Hip	Knee	Ankle	Hip	Knee	Ankle
Rectus femoris						
Semimembranosus						
Semitendinosus						
Biceps femoris long head						
Gastrocnemius						

14. The sciatic nerve comes off of which nerve roots? _____

On which side of the thigh is the sciatic nerve located?

_____ Anterior   _____ Posterior   _____ Medial   _____ Lateral

List the two nerves that the sciatic nerve divides into at the knee.

_____   _____

15. Describe the general pathway of the two divisions of the sciatic nerve as they descend from the knee to the foot.

_____

_____

16. Describe the general pathway of the femoral nerve and then identify the knee muscles it innervates.

_____

_____

17. During closed-chain knee extension, in which direction does the femur rotate on the tibia during terminal extension?

_____

_____

18. During an open kinetic chain knee extension activity, in which direction does the tibia rotate on the femur to achieve terminal extension?

_____

_____

19. What is the average Q angle? _____

Who has the larger Q angle?

Men: _____   Women: _____

■ ■ ■ Lab Activities

Student's Name _____ Date Due _____

1. Perform the motions of the knee joint with your partner.

A. Perform a motion and then your partner names the motion you performed.

B. Your partner states a motion and then you perform that motion.

2. Using question 7 from the worksheets for reference, for each of the motions available at the knee joint:

A. Place your open left hand in the correct orientation to represent the plane of a motion.

B. Place your right index finger to indicate the axis of that motion.

C. Enter the plane and axis for each motion in the following chart.

Motion	Plane	Axis
Flexion		
Extension		

3. Observe the amount of motion available at the knee joint in each plane. Estimate the degrees of knee flexion motion available by checking the box that most closely describes that amount of motion. (Do not measure with a goniometer.)

Motions	0°–45°	46°–90°	91°–135°	136°–180°
Flexion				

4. Passively move your partner through the available range of motion making note of the end feel. If possible repeat with several people. Review question 10 in the worksheets for the normal end feel.

A. Is your partner's end feel consistent with normal end feel?

_____

B. What structures create the end feel for this joint?

_____

_____

5. On the skeleton, anatomical models, and at least one partner, locate, palpate, and observe the following structures. The reference position is the anatomical position. Having pictures for reference is helpful when trying to find structures. Not all structures are palpable on your partner.

Tibia

Intercondylar eminence	A double-pointed prominence centered on the proximal surface of the tibia. It extends into the intercondyloid fossa of the femur. Cannot be palpated.
Medial condyle	The proximal medial aspect of the tibia. Palpate below the joint space on the medial surface.
Lateral condyle	The proximal lateral aspect of the tibia. Palpate below the joint space on the lateral surface.
Tibial plateau	The broad proximal end of the tibia including the medial and lateral condyles and the intercondylar eminence.

(Continued...)

Tibia *(continued)*

Tibial tuberosity	A protuberance on the proximal anterior midline of the tibia; the attachment for the patellar tendon. Palpate the patella and move your fingers distal to the insertion of the patellar tendon on the tibial tuberosity. *See Figure 17-16.*
Crest	The sharp anterior border along the ridge of the tibia. Palpate by moving your fingers distally from the tibial tuberosity along the crest. The crest is very superficial along most of its length. **FIGURE 18-7.** Palpating the crest of the tibia.
Medial malleolus	Enlarged distal medial surface of the tibia. Palpate on the medial surface of the ankle. **FIGURE 18-8.** Palpating the medial malleolus.

Fibula

Head	Enlarged proximal end of the fibula. Palpate on the lateral aspect of the knee. 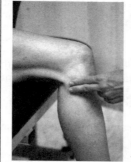 **FIGURE 18-9.** Palpating the head of the fibula.

(Continued...)

Fibula *(continued)*

Lateral malleolus	Enlarged distal lateral surface of the fibula. Palpate on the lateral aspect of the ankle. Note that the lateral malleolus extends further distally than the medial malleolus. 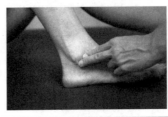 **FIGURE 18-10.** Palpating the lateral malleolus.

Other Structures

Patella	A triangular-shaped sesamoid bone on the anterior aspect of the knee. Palpate it on the anterior of the knee joint. With the person relaxed, move the patella in all directions making note of the amount of ROM. When the knee is flexed, this movement is not possible. **FIGURE 18-11.** Palpating the patella.
Posterior cruciate ligament	Located deep in the knee; attaches to the tibia posteriorly in the intercondylar area and runs in a superior and anterior direction to attach anteriorly on the medial condyle of the femur. It cannot be palpated.
Anterior cruciate ligament	Located deep in the knee; attaches to the tibia anteriorly in the intercondylar area and runs in a superior and posterior direction to attach posteriorly on the lateral condyle of the femur. It cannot be palpated.
Lateral collateral ligament	A cordlike structure located on the lateral aspect of the knee; attaches to the lateral condyle of the femur and the head of the fibula. With the knee in extension, palpate on the lateral surface of the knee by moving your fingers perpendicular to the weight-bearing surface of the tibia.
Medial collateral ligament	A flat broad ligament on the medial surface; attaches to the medial condyle of the femur and to the medial tibial condyle. Fibers of the medial meniscus attach to this ligament. Palpate it on the medial aspect of the knee.
Lateral meniscus	Located deep within the knee on the weight bearing surface of the lateral tibial condyle. It cannot be palpated.
Medial meniscus	Located deep within the knee on the weight bearing surface of the medial tibial condyle. Cannot be palpated.

(Continued...)

Calcaneus	Located on the posterior foot. 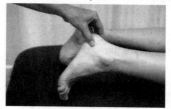 **FIGURE 18-12.** Palpating the calcaneus.

6. Use a disarticulated skeleton or anatomical model of the knee joint and apply the rules of joint arthrokinematics and the concave-convex rule to perform the following exercises.

   A. Underline the correct answer.

   The femur is: Concave   Convex.

   The tibia is: Concave   Convex.

   B. Move the tibia on the femur in all planes of motion.

   C. Observe the movement of the tibia on the femur. Circle the motions that you observed.

   Roll   Spin   Glide

   D. 1) Observe the movement of the distal end of the tibia in relation to the movement of the proximal end of the tibia as you move the tibia on the femur. Does the distal

      end of the tibia move in the _____ same or _____ opposite direction as the proximal end of the tibia?

      2) Observe the movement of the distal end of the femur in relation to the movement of the proximal end of the femur as you move the femur on the tibia. Does the

      distal end of the femur move in the _____ same or _____ opposite direction as the proximal end of the femur?

7. Locate the following on the skeleton, anatomical models, and at least one partner:

   A. Locate the origin and insertion of the muscle on the skeleton.

   B. Stretch a large rubber band taut by placing one end at the origin and the other end at the insertion of a muscle on the skeleton.

   C. Perform the motion that the muscle does and observe how the rubber band becomes less taut and shorter, similar to the muscle shortening as it contracts.

   D. Perform the opposite motion and observe how the rubber band becomes tauter and longer, similar to the muscle lengthening as it is being stretched.

   E. After locating the muscle on the skeleton, locate the muscle on your partner. The position described for locating the muscle on your partner is the manual muscle test position for a fair or better grade of muscle strength. Not all origins, insertions, and muscle bellies can be palpated on your partner.

   F. When possible, palpate the origin, insertion, and muscle belly of each muscle by:

      1) Placing your fingers on the origin and insertion, and asking your partner to contract the muscle.

      2) Moving your fingers from the origin and insertion over the contracting muscle.

      3) Asking your partner to relax the muscle and again moving your fingers from the origin to the insertion over the muscle.

      4) Note the differences between the contracting and relaxed muscles.

   G. In the following tables, the information needed to palpate each muscle is provided. The information includes position of the person, origin and insertion of the muscle, the line of pull of the muscle, the muscle's action, instructions to give to the person to make the muscle contract, and, finally, information on the best location to palpate the muscle.

      Review semimembranosus, semitendinosus, and biceps femoris in Chapter 17.

Sitting Position

RECTUS FEMORIS	Superficial on the anterior thigh.
	 FIGURE 18-13. Palpating the quadriceps muscle.
Position of person:	With hip and knee flexed.
Origin:	Anterior inferior iliac spine.
Insertion:	Tibial tuberosity via the patellar tendon.
Line of pull:	Vertical on the anterior surface of the thigh and over the knee joint.
Muscle action:	Knee extension, hip flexion.
Palpate:	Palpate along the midline of the thigh or at the patellar tendon. The origin can be isolated by palpating the tendon as it crosses the hip joint.
Instructions to person:	Straighten your knee.
VASTUS LATERALIS	Located superficial on the anterior lateral thigh. In Figure 18-13, thumb is over Vastus Lateralis.
	 FIGURE 18-14. Palpating muscle insertion at the tibial tuberosity.
Position of person:	With hip and knee flexed.
Origin:	Linea aspera.
Insertion:	Tibial tuberosity via the patellar tendon.
Line of pull:	Vertical on the anterior surface of the thigh and over the knee joint.
Muscle action:	Knee extension.
Palpate:	Palpate on the lateral portion of the thigh or at the patellar tendon.
Instructions to person:	Straighten your knee.

(Continued...)

Sitting Position (continued)

VASTUS MEDIALIS	Superficial on the anterior medial thigh. In Figure 18-13, fingers are over Vastus Medialis.
Position of person:	With hip and knee flexed.
Origin:	Linea aspera of the femur.
Insertion:	Tibial tuberosity via the patellar tendon.
Line of pull:	Vertical on the anterior surface of the thigh and over the knee joint.
Muscle action:	Knee extension.
Palpate:	Palpate along the medial portion of the thigh or the patellar tendon.
Instructions to person:	Straighten your knee.
VASTUS INTERMEDIALIS	Deep to the rectus femoris on the anterior thigh.
Position of person:	Hip and knee flexed.
Origin:	Anterior femur.
Insertion:	Tibial tuberosity via the patellar tendon.
Line of pull:	Vertical on the anterior surface of the thigh and over the knee joint.
Muscle action:	Knee extension.
Palpate:	Difficult to palpate directly because it is deep to the rectus femoris.
Instructions to person:	Straighten your knee.

Prone Position

SEMITENDINOSUS	A superficial muscle on the posterior medial aspect of the thigh. **See Figure 17-23.**
Position of person:	Hip and knee extended and in neutral alignment.
Origin:	Ischial tuberosity.
Insertion:	Proximal anterior medial tibia.
Line of pull:	Vertical on the posterior surface of the thigh and, the hip and knee joints.
Muscle action:	Hip extension and knee flexion.
Palpate:	Palpate on the posterior medial thigh. The long distal tendon is on the distal medial aspect of the thigh superficial to the attachment of the semimembranosus.
Instructions to person:	Lift your leg off the table keeping your knee bent.

(Continued...)

Prone Position *(continued)*

SEMIMEMBRANOSUS	Deep to the semitendinosus muscle and located on the posterior medial thigh. **See Figure 17-24.**
Position of person:	Hip and knee extended and in neutral alignment.
Origin:	Ischial tuberosity.
Insertion:	Posterior surface of the medial condyle of the tibia.
Line of pull:	Vertical on the posterior surface of the thigh and the hip and knee joints.
Muscle action:	Hip extension and knee flexion.
Palpate:	Palpate on the posterior medial thigh. Distinguishing between the semimembranosus and the semitendinosus can be difficult. The semimembranosus has a broad attachment on the posterior surface of the tibia deep to and on either side of the semitendinosus just above the knee joint.
Instructions to person:	Lift your leg off the table keeping your knee bent.
BICEPS FEMORIS	A superficial muscle on the posterior lateral thigh. **See Figure 17-25.**
Position of person:	Hip and knee extended and in neutral alignment.
Origin:	Long head: Ischial tuberosity. Short head: Lateral lip of the linea aspera of the femur.
Insertion:	Posterior proximal fibular head.
Line of pull:	Vertical on the posterior surface of the thigh and the hip and knee joints.
Muscle action:	Long head: Hip extension and knee flexion. Short head: Knee flexion.
Palpate:	Palpate on the posterior lateral thigh. The tendon is palpated on the distal lateral thigh at the knee joint.
Instructions to person:	Lift your leg off the table keeping your knee bent.
POPLITEUS	Deep to the gastrocnemius on the posterior proximal leg.
Position of person:	Hip and knee extended in neutral alignment.
Origin:	Lateral condyle of the femur.
Insertion:	Posterior medial condyle of the tibia.
Line of pull:	Diagonal on the posterior surface of the knee joint.
Muscle action:	Initiates knee flexion.
Palpate:	Cannot be palpated.
Instructions to person:	Flex your knee.

Standing Position

GASTROCNEMIUS	Superficial on the posterior of the leg.
	 FIGURE 18-15. Palpating the gastrocnemius.
Position of person:	Hip and knee extended, ankle in neutral.
Origin:	Posterior aspect of the medial and lateral condyles of the femur.
Insertion:	Via a common tendon onto the posterior aspect of the calcaneus.
Line of pull:	Vertical.
Muscle action:	Ankle plantar flexion.
Palpate:	Palpate on the posterior proximal medial and lateral aspects of the leg.
Instructions to person:	Rise up on your toes.

8. Referring to worksheets question 13, assume the positions that make the multijoint muscles:

    A. Lengthen simultaneously over all the joints they cross.

    B. Shorten simultaneously over all the joints they cross.

9. A break test is used when performing manual muscle testing for the good and normal grades. A break test is performed by placing the muscle in the mid-to-shorten range, and asking the patient to hold the part in that position as you apply resistance to "break" the hold. With your partner prone and the knee fully flexed, perform a break test of the knee flexors. Note that this may cause a muscle cramp if you hold it for too long. Repeat with your partner supine with the hip and knee flexed. Does the position of the hip, either flexed or extended, affect the strength of the hamstrings as knee flexors? Why?

    _____

    _____

10. With your partner standing, observe from the front to determine whether genu valgus and genu varus is present.

    A. Does your partner have?

       Genu valgus _____   Genu varus _____   Normal alignment _____

    B. With your partner supine, measure the Q angle using a goniometer. Place the axis of the goniometer over the midpoint of the patella. Align one arm of the goniometer with the AIIS and the other arm with the tibial tuberosity. How does your partner's Q angle compare to the normal range of the Q angle? _____

    _____

    C. Do the angles of the right and left lower extremities appear equal? _____

    _____

    D. The knee generally has a few degrees of motion in the sagittal plane beyond 0 degrees of extension. This motion is called hyperextension. Hyperextension is a normal amount of motion beyond zero allowed by ligament laxity. Knee hyperextension beyond 5° is considered genu recurvatum. Starting in the long sitting position, ask your partner to extend the knee as much as possible. Normally, the heel will rise less than an inch. Does your partner's heel come off the table and if so by how many inches?

    _____

    E. With your partner standing, observe from the side to determine if genu recurvatum is present.

11. What might be some of the effects on the weight-bearing surfaces of the knee when the line of gravity does not fall in the normal position through the knee joint because of varus, valgus, or recurvatum?

    _____

    _____

12. Diagram the lever that describes the activity at the knee joint when, starting in a standing position, a person lowers to a sitting position. Analyze the down motion.

    A. Draw a stick figure representing lowering to a sitting position.

    B. Draw arrows to indicate the direction of the movement, the direction of the pull of the muscle, and the direction of gravity.

    C. Label the arrow that represents force with an "F" and the arrow that represents resistance with an "R."

13. Analyze the activity of assuming sitting diagrammed in question 12 by answering the following questions:

   A. Which joint motion is being analyzed? _____

   B. Identify the "axis" of the motion: _____

   C. Would gravity cause the movement? _____

   D. Is the muscle acting to overcome gravity or slow down gravity? _____

   E. Is the "resistance" to the movement a muscle or gravity? _____

   F. Which major muscle group is the agonist? _____

   G. Which major muscle group is the antagonist? _____

   H. Is the agonist performing a concentric or an eccentric contraction? _____

   I. Is the antagonist active? _____

   J. Is this an open or closed kinetic chain activity? _____

14. Diagram the lever that describes the activity at the knee joint when a person returns to standing from a sitting position.

   A. Draw a stick figure representing rising to standing.

   B. Draw arrows to indicate the direction of the movement, the direction of the pull of the muscle, and the direction of gravity.

   C. Label the arrow that represents force with an "F" and the arrow that represents resistance with an "R."

15. Analyze the activity of assuming standing diagrammed in question 14 by answering the following questions:

   A. Which joint motion is being analyzed? _____

   B. Identify the "axis" of the motion: _____

   C. Would gravity cause the movement? _____

   D. Is the muscle acting to overcome gravity or slow down gravity? _____

   E. Is the "resistance" to the movement a muscle or gravity? _____

   F. Which major muscle group is the agonist? _____

G. Which major muscle group is the antagonist? _____

H. Is the agonist performing a concentric or an eccentric contraction? _____

I. Is the antagonist active? _____

J. Is this an open or closed kinetic chain activity? _____

■ ■ ■ Post-Lab Questions

Student's Name _____ Date Due _____

After you have completed the Worksheets and Lab Activities, answer the following questions without using your book or notes. When finished, check your answers.

1. In considering various impairments of the knee, you are reviewing the muscle(s) that attach distal to the knee and proximal to the pelvis. Name the multijoint muscles that cross the hip and knee.

   _____

   _____

2. In considering various impairments of the ankle, you are reviewing the muscle(s) that attach proximally on the femur and distally on the calcaneus. List the multijoint muscles that cross the knee and attach posteriorly on the calcaneus.

   _____

3. Which muscle of the hamstrings group does not cross the hip? _____

4. Which muscle of the quadriceps muscle group crosses the hip? _____

5. Starting at the tibial tuberosity and proceeding laterally around the knee, name, in order, the muscles that span the knee joint.

   _____

   _____

   _____

6. Describe the positions that make the hamstrings group actively insufficient.

   Hip _____   Knee _____

   Describe the positions that make the hamstrings group passively insufficient.

   Hip _____   Knee _____

7. Describe the positions that make the rectus femoris actively insufficient.

   Hip _____   Knee _____

   Describe the positions that make the rectus femoris passively insufficient.

   Hip _____   Knee _____

8. Why is the Q angle of women generally larger than the Q angle of men?

   _____

9. Identify the varus and valgus changes at the hips and knees in Figures 18-16 and 18-17.

A. Coxa _____   B. Genu _____

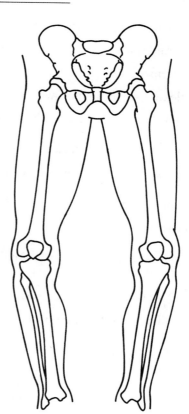

FIGURE 18-16. Coxa and genu varus and valgus.

A. Coxa _____   B. Genu _____

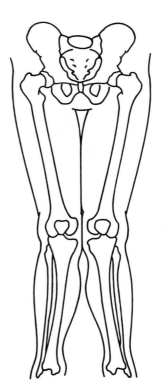

FIGURE 18-17. Coxa and genu varus and valgus.

10. Name the muscles that make up the pes anserine muscle group.

    _____

11. A. Knee extensors are located on which side of the knee?

    _____ Anterior   _____ Posterior

    B. Knee extensors are innervated by which nerve? _____

    C. Knee flexors are located on which side of the knee?

    _____ Anterior   _____ Posterior

12. A. The common name for the knee flexors that extend the hip is _____

    B. These muscles are innervated by which nerve? _____

13. A. What knee flexor is innervated by the common peroneal nerve? _____

    B. Is it located on the _____ medial or _____ lateral side of the posterior knee?

14. A. The popliteus muscle has its proximal attachment on which side of the posterior knee?

    _____ Medial   _____ Lateral

    B. The popliteus muscle is innervated by which nerve? _____

Ankle Joint and Foot

■ ■ ■ Worksheets

Student's Name _____ Date Due _____

Complete the following questions prior to the lab class.

1. Match the following terms with the appropriate descriptions.

   _____ Equinis   A. Abnormally high arch

   _____ Pes cavus   B. Valgus deformity of great toe

   _____ Pes planus   C. Hindfoot fixed in plantar flexion

   _____ Hallux valgus   D. Abnormally low arch

2. Match the parts of the foot with the bones that make up that part.

   _____ Hindfoot   A. Five metatarsals and all the phalanges

   _____ Midfoot   B. Talus and calcaneus

   _____ Forefoot   C. Navicular, cuboid, and three cuneiforms

3. On Figure 19-1:
   A. Identify the view
   B. Label the following bones and landmarks:

   Tarsals: Talus
                   Cuboid
                   Calcaneus: Sustentaculum tali
                   Cuneiforms: 1–3
                   Navicular: Tuberosity of the navicular

   Metatarsals: Base
                   Head

   Phalanges

   A _____ view   B _____ view   C _____ view

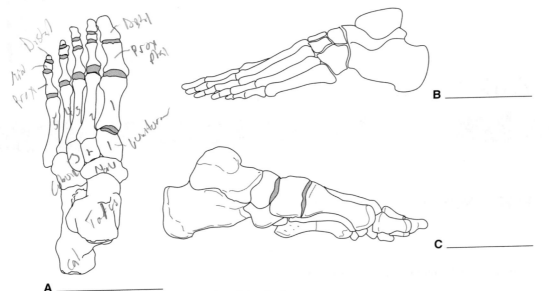

[handwritten annotations on foot: Distal, Distal, Mid, Prox pha, Prox pha, Prox, 3 4 5, 3 2 1, cuneiform, Cuboid, Nav, Talus, Cal]

B _____

C _____

A _____

FIGURE 19-1. Bones and landmarks of the foot.

4. On Figure 19-2, label the bones, landmarks, and ligaments.

BONES: Tibia   Fibula

LANDMARKS: Crest   Medial malleolus
                  Head   Lateral malleolus

LIGAMENTS:

Superior tibiofibular   Inferior tibiofibular   Interosseous membrane

[handwritten labels on leg diagram: Head of Fib., Crest, Interosseous Membrane, Fibula, Tibia, Medial malleolus, Lateral malleolus, Inferior Tibiofibular]

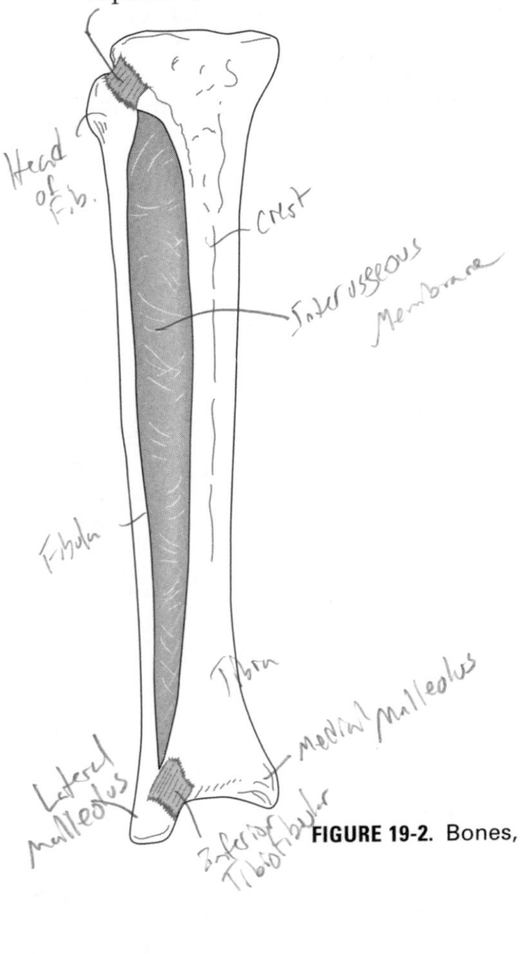

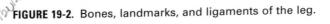

FIGURE 19-2. Bones, landmarks, and ligaments of the leg.

5. On Figures 19-3 and 19-4, label the joints and identify bones that make up the joints.

Talocrural joint
Subtalar joint
Transverse tarsal joint

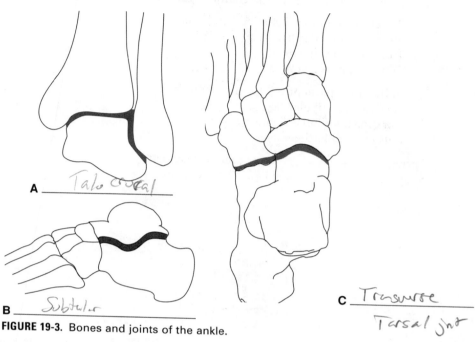

A ____Talo crural____

B ____Subtalar____

C ____Transverse Tarsal jnt____

FIGURE 19-3. Bones and joints of the ankle.

Metatarsophalangeal (MTP), Tarsometatarsal (TM)
Interphalangeal: proximal (PIP), distal (DIP), and interphalangeal (IP)

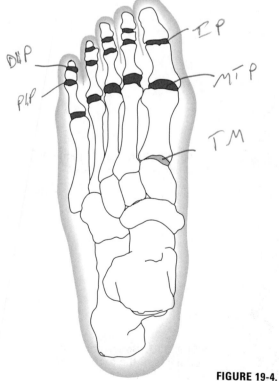

FIGURE 19-4. Bones and joints of the foot.

6. Label the bones and ligaments on Figures 19-5, 19-6, and 19-7.

BONES: Cuboid   Metatarsals   Navicular   Tibia
            Talus   Calcaneus   Cuneiforms   Fabula

LIGAMENTS: Label the four parts of the Deltoid ligament

        Posterior tibiotalar ligament
        Anterior tibiotalar ligament
        Tibionavicular ligament
        Tibiocalcaneal ligament

      Label the three parts of the Lateral ligament
        Posterior talofibular ligament
        Anterior talofibular ligament
        Calcaneofibular ligament

      Spring ligament   Long plantar ligament
      Short plantar ligament Plantar aponeurosis

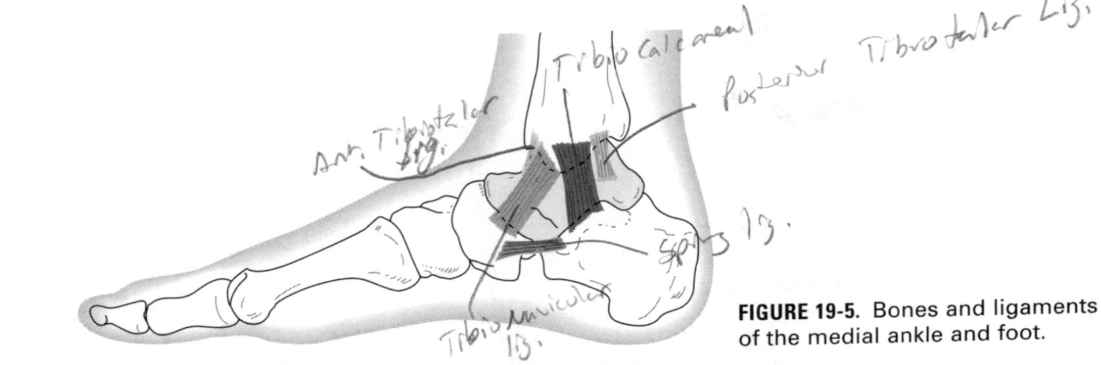

FIGURE 19-5. Bones and ligaments of the medial ankle and foot.

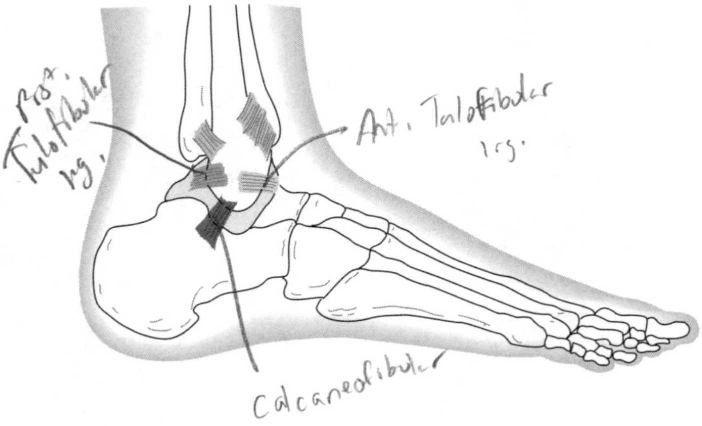

FIGURE 19-6. Bones and ligaments of the lateral ankle and foot.

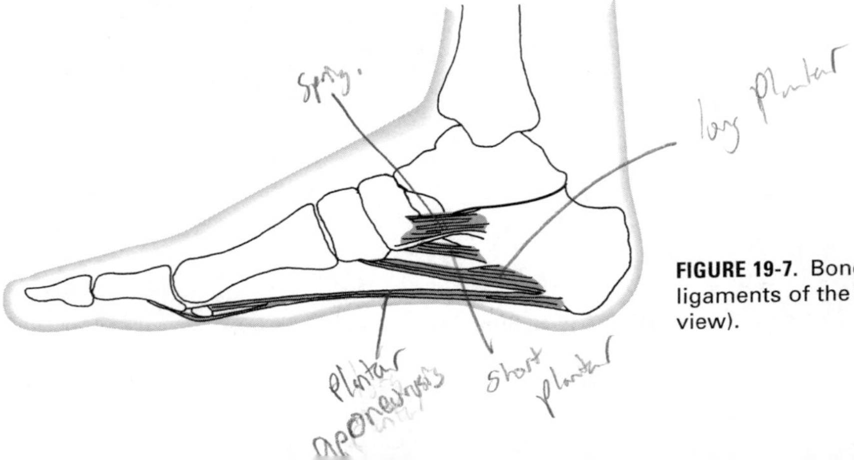

FIGURE 19-7. Bones and inferior ligaments of the foot (medial view).

7. Label the arches, and bones making up those arches, on Figures 19-8 A, B, and C.

  ARCHES: Medial longitudinal arch   Lateral longitudinal arch
            Transverse arch

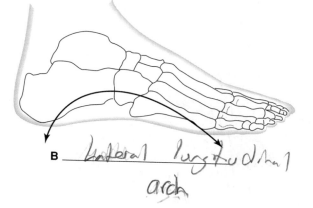

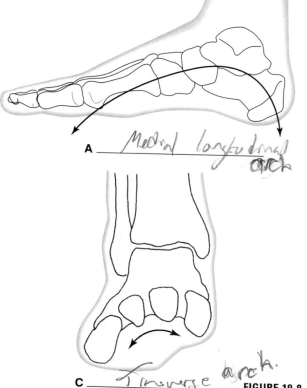

A _Medial longitudinal arch_

B _Lateral longitudinal arch_

C _Transverse arch._

FIGURE 19-8. Arches of the ankle and foot.

8. On Figures 19-9 through 19-16:

  A. Label the origin and insertion of the muscles listed.

  B. Join the origin and insertion to show the line of pull.

  Gastrocnemius
  Soleus
  Plantaris

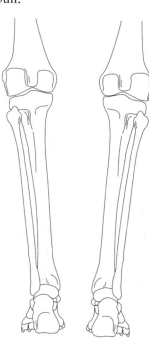

FIGURE 19-9. Gastrocnemius, soleus, and plantaris.

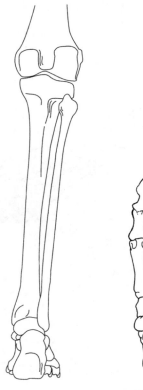

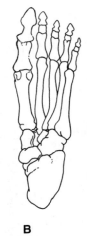

A

B

FIGURE 19-10. *(A)* and *(B)* Tibialis posterior.

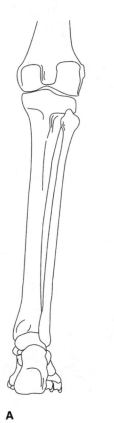

A

B

FIGURE 19-11. *(A)* and *(B)* Flexor hallucis longus.

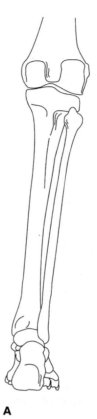
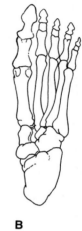

FIGURE 19-12. *(A)* and *(B)* Flexor digitorum longus.

A   **B**

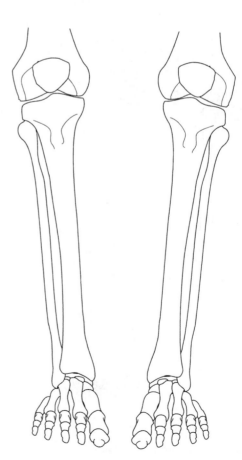

FIGURE 19-13. Tibialis anterior and extensor hallucis longus.

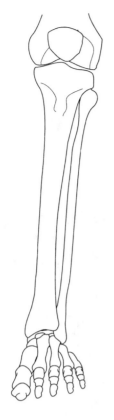

FIGURE 19-14. Extensor digitorum longus.

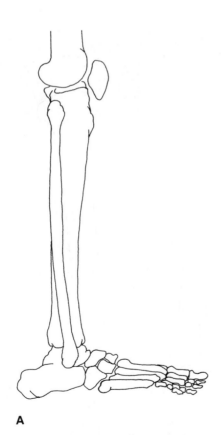

A

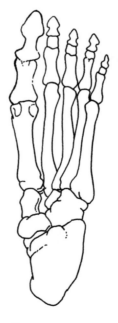

B

FIGURE 19-15. Peroneus longus.

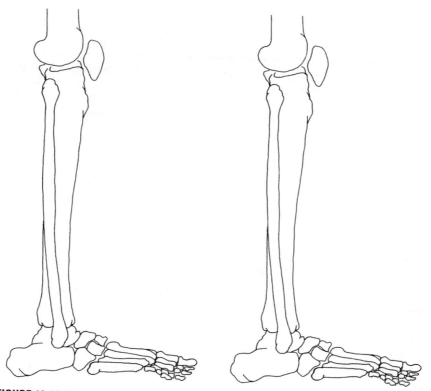

FIGURE 19-16. Peroneus brevis and peroneus tertius.

9. For each of the following joints, give the following information:

Joint	Shape	Degrees of Freedom	Motions
Talocrural			
Metatarsophalangeal			
Interphalangeal of great toe			

10. For each of the following joints, provide the close-packed position and the loose-packed position. (Refer to Chapter 4.)

Joint	Close-Packed	Loose-Packed
Talocrural		
Subtalar		
Transverse tarsal		

11. For each of the following joints, describe the normal end feel. (Refer to Chapter 4 for descriptions.)

Joints	Bony	Capsular	Soft Tissue Approximation
Talocrural			
Subtalar			
Metatarsophalangeal of great toe			

12. Match each ligament and structure listed below with the appropriate function or characteristic. Use each answer once.

_____ Deltoid ligament

_____ Medial longitudinal arch

_____ Spring ligament

_____ Plantar aponeurosis

_____ Transverse arch

_____ Lateral ligament

A. Three parts, each with an insertion on the fibula

B. Located on the medial side, triangular in shape

C. Runs from side to side at the distal row of tarsals.

D. Supports the medial side of the longitudinal arch

E. The talus is the keystone

F. Supports both longitudinal arches

13. For each muscle listed check the motions for which it is a prime mover.

Muscle	Plantar Flexion	Dorsiflexion	Eversion	Inversion	Flexion	Extension
Gastrocnemius						
Soleus						
Plantaris						
Tibialis posterior						
Flexor hallucis longus						
Flexor digitorum longus						
Tibialis anterior						
Extensor hallucis longus						
Extensor digitorum longus						
Peroneus longus						
Peroneus brevis						
Peroneus tertius						

14. List the multijoint muscles, the joints they cross, and the positions that simultaneously lengthen or shorten them over all the joints they cross.

Muscle	Lengthened Position				Shortened Position			
	Knee	Ankle	Foot	MP, IP	Knee	Ankle	Foot	MP, IP
Gastrocnemius								
Soleus								
Plantaris								
Tibialis posterior								
Flexor hallucis longus								
Flexor digitorum longus								
Tibialis anterior								
Extensor hallucis longus								
Extensor digitorum								
Peroneus longus								
Peroneus brevis								
Peroneus tertius								

■ ■ ■ Lab Activities

Student's Name _____ Date Due _____

1. Perform the motions of the ankle and foot joint with your partner.
   A. Perform a motion and then your partner names the motion you performed.
   B. Your partner states a motion and then you perform that motion.

2. Observe the amount of motion available at each joint.

   For each of the motions available at each joint, estimate the degrees of motion available by checking the box that *most closely* describes that amount of motion. (Do not measure with a goniometer.)

Motions	0°–45°	46°–90°	91°–135°	136°–180°
Dorsiflexion				
Plantar flexion				
MTP flexion				
MTP extension				
MTP abduction of the great toe				

3. Passively move your partner through the available range of motion of the ankle joint noting end feel. If possible repeat with several people. Review question 11 in the worksheets for the normal end feel.

   A. Is your partner's end feel consistent with normal end feel? _____

   B. What structures create the end feel for this joint?

   _____

   _____

4. On the skeleton, anatomical models, and at least one partner, locate, palpate, and observe the following structures. The reference position is the anatomical position. Having pictures for reference is helpful when trying to find structures. Not all structures can be palpated on your partner.

Tarsal Bones and Landmarks

Calcaneus	The largest and most posterior tarsal bone; also called the heel. Palpate by grasping the heel. 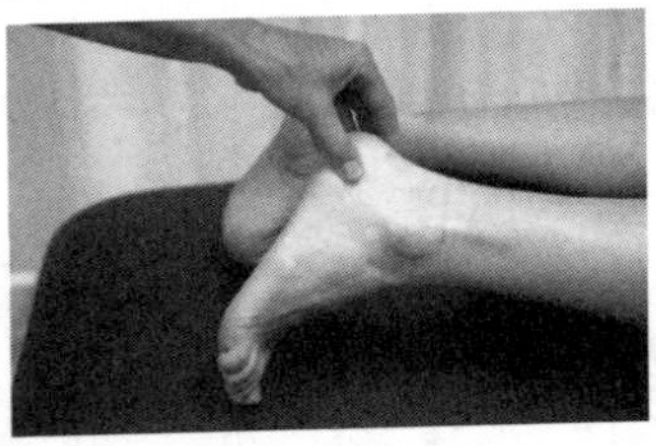 **FIGURE 19-17.** Palpating the calcaneus.
Calcaneal tuberosity	The rounded area on the posterior surface.
Sustentaculum tali	A small protuberance on the proximal medial side of the calcaneus. Palpate the medial malleolus, then move your finger distal about two finger-widths. The tip may be more distinct with the ankle passively inverted.
Talus	Between the tibia and calcaneus. With the foot in plantar flexion, the talus can be palpated on the dorsum of the foot distal to the tibia. The talus can also be palpated between the navicular tuberosity and the medial malleolus. 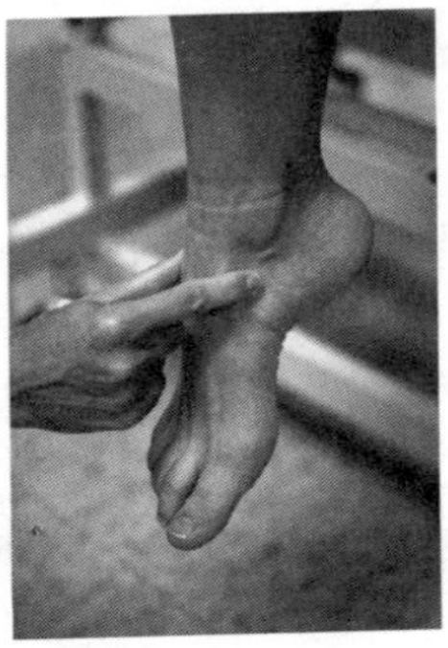 **FIGURE 19-18.** Palpating the talus.

(Continued...)

Navicular	Located on the medial side of the foot between the talus and the cuneiforms. Palpate on the dorsum and medial side of the foot. 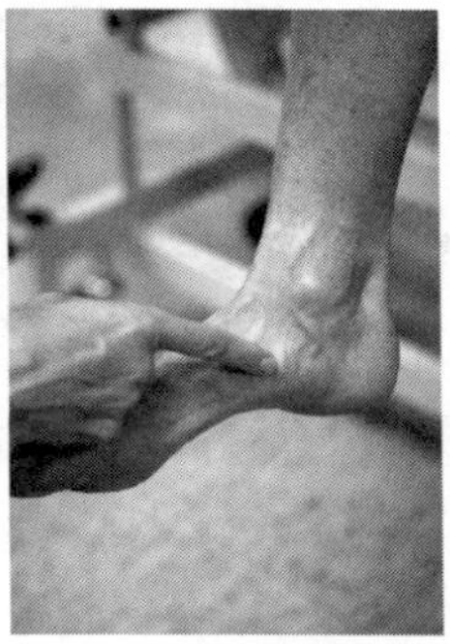 **FIGURE 19-19.** Palpating the navicular.
Tuberosity of the navicular	A protuberance on the medial surface of the navicular. Palpate on the medial side of the foot distal to the medial malleolus. Palpation is easier with the foot inverted because the tuberosity becomes more pronounced.
Cuboid	Located on the lateral side of the foot between the calcaneus and the metatarsals. Palpate its flat surface on the lateral side of the foot. Place one finger on the base of the fifth metatarsal and one finger on the lateral malleolus. The cuboid is located between the two fingers just proximal to the fifth metatarsal. 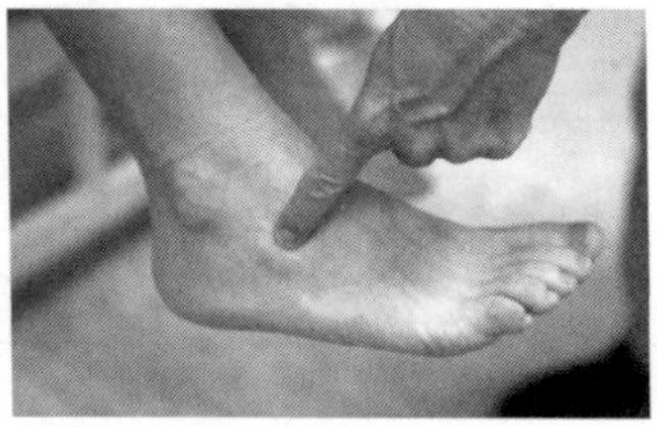 **FIGURE 19-20.** Palpating the cuboid.
Cuneiforms: 1–3	The first cuneiform is located on the medial side of the foot, the second is lateral to the first, and the third is between the second and the cuboid. The cuneiforms are between the navicular and the metatarsals. Palpate starting from the medial side of the foot and move laterally. Locate the first metatarsal and slide your finger proximal to the indentation of the first TMT joint. The first cuneiform is just proximal. Move your finger lateral along the dorsal surface to the second and third cuneiforms. 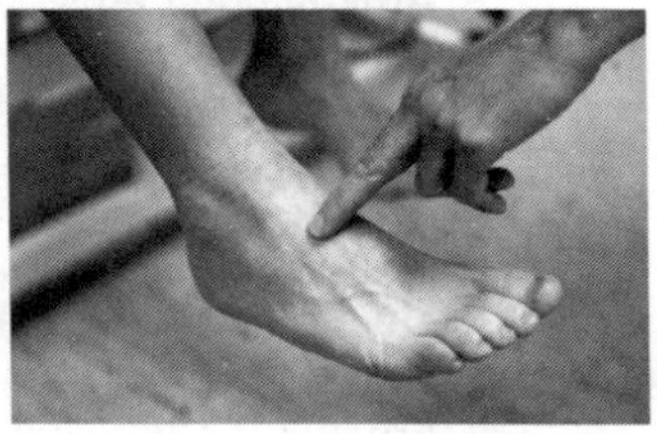 **FIGURE 19-21.** Palpating the cuneiforms.

Metatarsals

1–5	Located between the tarsals (cuneiforms and cuboid) and the phalanges. Palpate between the tarsals, and the phalanges from medial to lateral.

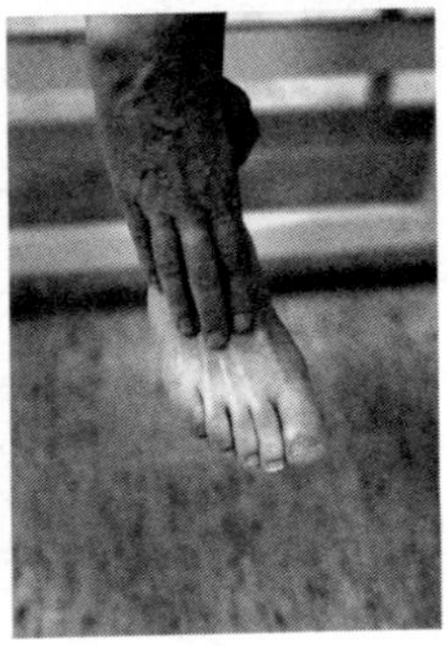

FIGURE 19-22. Palpating the metatarsals.

Base	Proximal end of each metatarsal.
Head	Distal end of each metatarsal.
First	Thickest and shortest, located on medial side of the foot. It articulates with the great toe.
Second	The longest; articulates with the second cuneiform and the second toe.
Third	Articulates with the third cuneiform and the third toe.
Fourth	Articulates with the cuboid and the fourth toe.
Fifth	Articulates with the cuboid and the fifth toe.

Phalanges

Great toe (lst)	Two—proximal, distal.
Lesser toes (2nd–5th)	Three each—proximal, middle, distal.

Joints

Superior tibiofibular	Articulation between the head of the fibula and the proximal posterior lateral aspect of the tibia. Palpate just above the fibular head.
Inferior tibiofibular	Articulation between the distal tibia and the distal fibula on the lateral side of the ankle. Palpate an indentation just medial to the midpart of the lateral malleolus.
Talocrural or talotibial or ankle	Articulation between the tibia and talus. First palpate the medial and lateral malleoli, while moving the foot in the sagittal plane. Next, move the fingers from the malleoli to the midpoint between the malleoli as the joint is being moved to palpate the talus.
Subtalar or talocalcaneal	Articulation of the inferior surface of the talus with the superior surface of the calcaneus. Difficult to palpate.

(Continued...)

Transverse tarsal or midtarsal	Articulations of the anterior surface of the talus and calcaneus with the navicular and cuboid, respectively. Palpate slightly anterior between the navicular tuberosity and the medial malleolus, and between the cuboid and lateral malleolus.
Tarsometatarsal	Articulations of the cuneiforms and cuboid with the metatarsals.
Metatarsophalangeal	Articulations between the respective metatarsals and proximal phalanges of the toes.
Interphalangeal	Articulations between the proximal and distal phalanges of the great toe and between the proximal and middle and middle and distal phalanges of the lesser toes.

Ligaments and Other Structures

Joint capsule	Surrounds the ankle joint and is reinforced by ligaments. Cannot be palpated.
Deltoid ligament: tibionavicular; tibiocalcaneal; posterior tibiotalar; and anterior tibiotalar	Triangular ligament on the medial side of the ankle joint; attachments are a narrow proximal attachment on the tip of the medial malleolus and broader distal attachment on the talus, navicular, and calcaneus. Palpate on the medial side of the foot just distal to the medial malleolus. Move your finger anterior and posterior as the foot is moved in eversion and inversion.
Lateral ligament: anterior talofibular; posterior talofibular; and calcaneofibular	On lateral side of the ankle joining the lateral malleolus to the talus and calcaneus. The weak anterior talofibular ligament attaches the lateral malleolus to the talus anteriorly. The stronger posterior talofibular ligament is horizontal connecting the lateral malleolus to the talus posteriorly. The calcaneofibular ligament is located between the anterior and posterior talofibular ligaments and is a long, fairly vertical, ligament joining the lateral malleolus to the calcaneus. Palpate on the lateral side of the foot distal to the lateral malleolus to feel the calcaneofibular ligament. Move your fingers anteriorly and posteriorly as the foot is moved in inversion and eversion to feel the anterior and posterior talofibular ligaments respectively.
Medial longitudinal arch	A proximal-distal arch on the medial border of the foot consisting of the calcaneus, talus, navicular, three cuneiforms, and first three metatarsals. Observe the medial border of the foot both in weight-bearing and non–weight-bearing.
Lateral longitudinal arch	A proximal-distal arch on the lateral border of the foot consisting of the calcaneus, cuboid, and third and fourth metatarsals. Observe the lateral border of the foot. Note that there appears to be very little visible arch.
Transverse arch	A side-to-side arch in the midfoot consisting of the three cuneiforms and the cuboid. To accentuate the arch, press up in the middle of the plantar surface of the foot over the heads of the metatarsals. A callous in this area tends to be indicative of a low transverse arch.
Spring ligament or plantar calcaneonavicular	A short, wide ligament on the medial side supporting the medial longitudinal arch. Attaches from the calcaneus to the navicular. Palpate deeply just posterior to the navicular tuberosity. Roll your finger vertically over the ligament.

(Continued...)

Ligaments and Other Structures *(continued)*

Long plantar ligament	Superficial. Attaches to the calcaneus and runs forward to attach on the cuboid and bases of the third, fourth, and fifth metatarsals. Supports the lateral longitudinal arch. Difficult to separate from the short plantar ligament when palpating.
Short plantar ligament	Deep to the long plantar ligament on the lateral side of the foot; attaches to the calcaneus and cuboid. Difficult to separate from long plantar ligament when palpating.
Plantar aponeurosis	Superficial on the plantar surface of the foot. It supports both longitudinal arches; attaches to the calcaneus and the proximal phalanges. Palpate on the plantar surface anterior to the calcaneus while hyperextending the toes.

5. Using a skin pencil or colored yarn, follow the paths of the major nerves that serve the lower extremity from the lumbosacral plexus. Note where the nerves are superficial and where they are deep. Refer to Chapter 6 "The Nervous System."

Nerves to trace: femoral, obturator, sciatic, tibial, medial and lateral plantar, common peroneal, and superficial and deep peroneal.

6. Use a disarticulated skeleton or anatomical model of the ankle joint and apply the rules of joint arthrokinematics and the concave-convex rule to perform the following exercises.

A. Move the talus on the tibia in all planes of motion.

B. Observe the movement of the distal bone on the proximal bone. Circle the motions that you observed.

Roll　　　　　　Spin　　　　　　Glide

C. Observe the movement of the distal end of the tibia in relation to the movement of the proximal end of the tibia as you move the tibia on the talus. Does the distal end

of the tibia move in the _____ same direction or _____ opposite direction of the proximal end of the tibia?

7. Locate the following on the skeleton, anatomical models and at least one partner:

A. Locate the origin and insertion of the muscle on the skeleton.

B. Stretch a large rubber band taut by placing one end at the origin and the other end at the insertion of a muscle on the skeleton.

C. Perform the motion that the muscle does and observe how the rubber band becomes less taut and shorter, similar to the muscle shortening as it contracts.

D. Perform the opposite motion and observe how the rubber band becomes more taut and longer, similar to the muscle lengthening as it is being stretched.

E. After locating the muscle on the skeleton, locate the muscle on your partner. The position described for locating the muscle on your partner is the manual muscle test position for a fair or better grade of muscle strength. Not all origins, insertions, and muscle bellies can be palpated on your partner.

F. When possible, palpate the origin, insertion, and muscle belly of each muscle by:

　1) Placing your fingers on the origin and insertion, and asking your partner to contract the muscle.

　2) Moving your fingers from the origin and insertion over the contracting muscle.

　3) Asking your partner to relax the muscle and again moving your fingers from the origin to the insertion over the muscle.

　4) Note the difference between the contracting and relaxed muscle.

G. In the following tables, the information needed to palpate each muscle is provided. The information includes position of the person, origin and insertion of the muscle, the line of pull of the muscle, the muscle's action, instructions to give to the person to make the muscle contract, and, finally, information on the best location to palpate the muscle.

Standing Position

GASTROCNEMIUS	Located superficially on the posterior leg.
	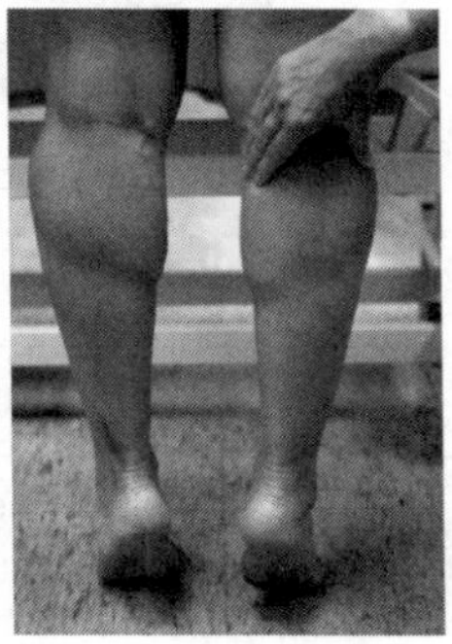 FIGURE 19-23. Palpating the gastrocnemius.
Position of person:	With ankle in neutral or a few degrees of dorsiflexion and the knee in extension.
Origin:	Medial head: Posterior on medial condyle of femur. Lateral head: Posterior on lateral condyle of femur.
Insertion:	Posterior calcaneus.
Line of pull:	Vertical.
Muscle action:	Ankle plantar flexion, knee flexion.
Palpate:	Posterior aspect of the leg in the upper-third region.
Instructions to person:	Rise up on your toes.
SOLEUS	Located deep to the gastrocnemius on the posterior leg.
Position of person:	With ankle in neutral or a few degrees of dorsiflexion and the knee in partial flexion.
Origin:	Posterior tibia and fibula.
Insertion:	Posterior calcaneus.
Line of pull:	Vertical.
Muscle action:	Ankle plantar flexion.
Palpate:	Distal to, and on both sides of, the muscle belly of the gastrocnemius.
Instructions to person:	Keeping your knee slightly bent, rise up on your toes.

Sitting Position

TIBIALIS POSTERIOR	Muscle belly is deep to the soleus and gastrocnemius; tendon passes posterior to medial malleolus and around the medial side of the foot to its insertions. **FIGURE 19-24.** Palpating the tibialis posterior.
Position of person:	Foot unsupported.
Origin:	Interosseous membrane, adjacent tibia and fibula.
Insertion:	Navicular and most tarsals and metatarsals.
Line of pull:	Vertical on the posterior surface of the lower leg and ankle.
Muscle action:	Inversion; assists with plantar flexion.
Palpate:	The tendon can be palpated behind the medial malleolus in the space between the malleolus and the Achilles tendon. The tendon can also be palpated between the medial malleolus and the navicular. It is difficult to distinguish between the tendons of the tibialis posterior, flexor hallucis longus, and flexor digitorum longus. Palpating distal to the medial malleolus while moving the ankle and toes can assist in differentiating among these tendons.
Instructions to person:	Point your toes down and in.
FLEXOR HALLUCIS LONGUS	Muscle belly is deep to the soleus and gastrocnemius; tendon passes posterior to the medial malleolus and around the medial side of the foot to its insertions (Fig. 19-25). **FIGURE 19-25.** Palpating the flexor hallucis longus.
Position of person:	Foot supported in neutral.
Origin:	Posterior fibula and interosseous membrane.
Insertion:	Distal phalange of the great toe.
Line of pull:	Vertical on the posterior surface of the lower leg and ankle.

(Continued...)

Sitting Position _(continued)_

Muscle action:	Flexes the great toe at the MP and IP joints; assists inversion and plantar flexion of the ankle.
Palpate:	The tendon is palpated posterior and inferior to the medial malleolus and on the medial side of the foot at the head of the great toe distal to the medial malleolus (same as with the tibialis posterior).
Instructions to person:	Curl your toes.
FLEXOR DIGITORUM LONGUS	Muscle belly is deep to the soleus and gastrocnemius; tendon passes posterior to the medial malleolus and around the medial side of the foot to its insertions.
Position of person:	With ankle in neutral.
Origin:	Posterior tibia.
Insertion:	Distal phalanges of the four lesser toes.
Line of pull:	Vertical on the posterior surface of the lower leg and ankle.
Muscle action:	Flexes the four lesser toes and assists in ankle inversion and plantar flexion.
Palpate:	Posterior to the medial malleolus and along the medial aspect of the foot (same as with tibialis posterior).
Instructions to person:	Curl your toes.
TIBIALIS ANTERIOR	Located superficially on the anterior lateral leg. **FIGURE 19-26.** Palpating the tibialis anterior.
Position of person:	Ankle in neutral.
Origin:	Lateral tibia and interosseous membrane.
Insertion:	First cuneiform and metatarsal.
Line of pull:	Vertical on the anterior surface of the lower leg and ankle.
Muscle action:	Ankle inversion and dorsiflexion.
Palpate:	Palpate the belly on the anterior lateral aspect of the tibia by identifying the tibial shaft, and moving your fingers just lateral. Palpate the tendon as it crosses anteriorly to the medial side of the ankle.
Instructions to person:	Bring your foot up and in.

(Continued...)

Sitting Position *(continued)*

EXTENSOR HALLUCIS LONGUS	Muscle belly is deep to the tibialis anterior and extensor digitorum longus muscles; tendon is on the dorsum of the foot. **FIGURE 19-27.** Palpating the extensor hallucis longus.
Position of person:	Ankle in neutral.
Origin:	Anterior fibula and interosseous membrane.
Insertion:	Distal phalange of the great toe.
Line of pull:	Vertical on the anterior surface of the lower leg and ankle.
Muscle action:	Extends the great toe; assists in ankle inversion and dorsiflexion.
Palpate:	Anterior as it crosses the ankle and on the dorsum of the foot to the insertion.
Instructions to person:	Straighten your great toe pointing it to the ceiling.
EXTENSOR DIGITORUM LONGUS	Muscle belly is deep to the tibialis anterior. **FIGURE 19-28.** Palpating the extensor digitorum longus.
Position of person:	Ankle in neutral.
Origin:	Anterior fibula, interosseous membrane, and anterior lateral tibia.
Insertion:	Dorsum of the distal phalanges of the four lesser toes.
Line of pull:	Vertical on the anterior surface of the lower leg and ankle.
Muscle action:	Extends four lesser toes, assists in ankle dorsiflexion.
Palpate:	Palpate and observe the four tendons on the dorsum of the foot.
Instructions to person:	Straighten your toes and point them to the ceiling.

(Continued...)

PERONEUS LONGUS	Located on the anterior lateral side of the leg, partially covered by the tibialis anterior and superficial to the other peroneal muscles.
	FIGURE 19-29. Palpating the peroneus longus. The examiner's left index finger is over the origin and the right fingers are over the tendon.
Position of person:	Ankle and foot in neutral.
Origin:	Proximal lateral fibula and interosseous membrane.
Insertion:	Plantar surface of the first cuneiform and metatarsal.
Line of pull:	Vertical on the lateral surface of the lower leg and ankle.
Muscle action:	Ankle eversion; assists in plantar flexion.
Palpate:	The muscle belly can be palpated on the lateral side distal to the head of the fibula and the lateral malleolus. The tendon is palpated posterior to the lateral malleolus before going deep on the plantar surface of the foot.
Instructions to person:	Point your toes and move your foot to the outside.
PERONEUS BREVIS	The muscle belly is deep to the peroneus longus on the distal lateral leg.
	FIGURE 19-30. Palpating the tendon of the peroneus brevis.
Position of person:	Ankle and foot in neutral.
Origin:	Distal lateral fibula.
Insertion:	Base of the fifth metatarsal.
Line of pull:	Vertical on the lateral surface of the lower leg and ankle.
Muscle action:	Ankle eversion; assists in plantar flexion.
Palpate:	The muscle belly is palpated on the distal lateral fibula but cannot be distinguished from the peroneus longus. The tendon can be palpated inferior to the lateral malleolus as it goes to its insertion on the base of the fifth metatarsal.
Instructions to person:	Move your foot to the outside.

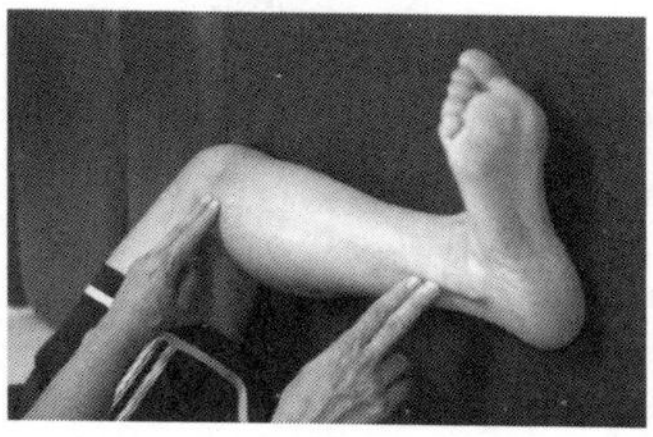

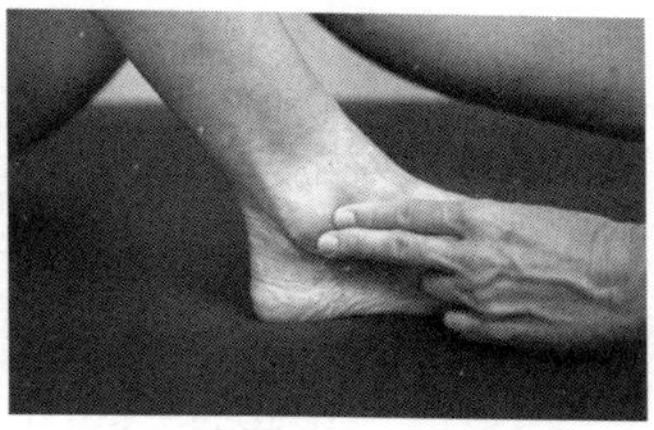

(Continued...)

Sitting Position *(continued)*

PERONEUS TERTIUS	The muscle belly is deep to the peroneus longus and extensor digitorum longus on the distal anterior lateral leg.
Position of person:	Ankle and foot in neutral.
Origin:	Distal medial fibula.
Insertion:	Base of the fifth metatarsal.
Line of pull:	Vertical on the lateral side of the ankle.
Muscle action:	Assists in ankle eversion and dorsiflexion.
Palpate:	The tendon is palpated from anterior to the lateral malleolus on the dorsum of the foot to the insertion on the head of the fifth metatarsal. It is not easily seen or palpated on all individuals. Do not confuse it with the tendon of the extensor digitorum longus.
Instructions to person:	Point your toes up and out.

Prone Position

PLANTARIS	Located deep to the lateral head of the gastrocnemius.
Position of person:	With ankle in neutral and the knee flexed.
Origin:	Posterior lateral condyle of the femur.
Insertion:	Posterior calcaneus.
Line of pull:	Vertical on the posterior side of the lower leg and ankle.
Muscle action:	Assists in ankle plantar flexion.
Palpate:	Locate the fibular head. Move your fingers medially into the Popliteal space. Moving your fingers slightly proximal moves you away from the heads of the gastrocnemius. Press deeply.
Instructions to person:	Point your toes.

8. List the muscles in each of the following groups.

Muscle Group	Muscles
Superficial posterior	
Deep posterior	
Anterior	
Lateral	

9. Describe the orientation of the malleoli in relation to one another.

_____

10. What position of the knee effects range of motion at the ankle? Explain why.

_____

11. Stand with your back no more than 6 inches from a wall. Lean backward from your ankles until your shoulders touch the wall. Return to standing erect.

A. What ankle motion allows you to lean backward?

_____

B. Which ankle muscle(s) controls the movement as you lean backward?

_____

C. What type of muscle contraction controls the lean backward motion?

_____

D. What ankle motion allows you to return to an erect standing position?

_____

E. Which ankle muscle group controls the return to erect standing motion?

_____

F. What type of muscle contraction controls the return to erect standing motion?

_____

G. Is this an open- or closed-chain activity?

_____

H. What term is used to describe muscle action that occurs when the origin moves rather than the insertion?

_____

12. The anatomical axes of the tibia and calcaneus may form a very slight angle. This angle is measured by aligning a goniometer over the posterior midline of the tibia and calcaneus with the pivot at the ankle joint.

Calcaneal varus is a decreased angle resulting in the calcaneus appearing to be inverted.

Calcaneal valgus is an increased angle resulting in the calcaneus appearing to be everted.

A. Observe your partner's tibial calcaneal angle in the standing position.

B. Is the observed angle:

_____ Normal   _____ Decreased   _____ Increased

C. Are the right and left angles the

_____ Same   _____ Different

D. Observe the heels of your partner's shoes for the part of the heel that is most worn. Does this correlate with the position of the calcaneus?

13. Dip the sole of one foot in a tub of water and then briefly step on a piece of paper, for example a paper towel. Observe the water mark your foot left on the paper.

    A. Describe the parts of your foot that contacted the supporting surface.

    _____

    B. Does the water mark indicate your foot is in

    _____ Pes cavus   _____ Pes planus

14. Analyze the activity of the right ankle when descending stairs leading with the left foot. To perform this activity start facing down the stairs with both feet on the top step. Lower your left foot to the next lower stair.

    A. Which joint motion is being analyzed? _____

    B. Identify the "axis" of the motion: _____

    C. Is this motion with gravity or against gravity? _____

    D. Is the muscle acting to _____ slow down gravity _____ overcome gravity?

    E. Thus gravity is the _____ force _____ resistance and muscle is the _____ force

       _____ resistance.

    F. Which major muscle group is the agonist? _____

    G. Is the agonist performing a concentric or an eccentric contraction? _____

    H. Is this an open or closed kinetic chain activity? _____

15. Analyze the activity of the right ankle when ascending stairs leading with the right foot. To perform this activity start facing up the stairs with both feet at the bottom step. Place your right foot on the first stair and lift your body up using the right leg.

    A. Which joint motion is being analyzed? _____

    B. Identify the "axis" of the motion: _____

    C. Is this motion with gravity or against gravity? _____

    D. Is the muscle acting to _____ slow down gravity _____ overcome gravity?

    E. Thus gravity is the _____ force _____ resistance and muscle is the _____ force

       _____ resistance

    F. Which major muscle group is the agonist? _____

    G. Is the agonist performing a concentric or an eccentric contraction? _____

    H. Is this an open or closed kinetic chain activity? _____

■ ■ ■ Post-Lab Questions

After you have completed the Worksheets and Lab Activities, answer the following questions without using your book or notes. When finished, check your answers.

Student's Name _____ Date Due _____

1. List the motions and prime movers for each of the following joints.

Joints	Motions	Muscles
Ankle		
Subtalar		
Metatarsophalangeal of great toe		

2. List the attachments for the following ankle and foot ligaments.

Ligament	Proximal Attachments	Distal Attachments
Deltoid		
Spring		
Lateral		
Long plantar		

3. For the following ankle and foot ligaments, give the function.

Ligament	Function
Deltoid	
Lateral	
Long plantar	
Plantar aponeurosis	

4. Indicate the relationship of the peroneal muscles' tendons to the lateral malleolus.

Muscle	Anterior	Posterior
Peroneus longus		
Peroneus brevis		
Peroneus tertius		

5. In general, which nerves innervate the following muscle groups?

Muscle Group	Nerve
Dorsiflexors	
Plantar flexors	
Evertors	

6. Starting at the anterior medial aspect of the ankle, name in order the muscles/tendons that cross the ankle as you move laterally around the ankle joint.

_____

_____

7. What is the effect of toe extension on the longitudinal arches of the foot?

_____

8. Give the keystone bone for the arches of the foot.

Arch	Keystone Bone
Medial longitudinal	
Lateral longitudinal	
Transverse	

9. List the bones that make up each of the following parts of the foot.

Foot Part	Bones
Hindfoot	
Midfoot	
Forefoot	

10. Which nerve is superficial at the head of the fibula?

_____

11. Give the prime movers and the muscles that must act to neutralize undesired motions when only the motion listed is to be performed.

Motion	Prime Mover	Neutralizer
Dorsiflexion		
Inversion		
Eversion		

12. Why might a person have less ankle dorsiflexion when the knee is extended?

13. The sustentaculum tali is located on which bone? _____

14. What is the function of the sustentaculum tali? _____

Clinical Kinesiology and Anatomy of the Body

Posture

■ ■ ■ **Worksheets**

Student's Name _____ Date Due _____

Complete the following questions prior to the lab class.

1. Define the following terms:

   Primary curve _____

   Secondary curves _____

   Antigravity muscles _____

   Postural sway _____

2. When performing a standing postural assessment from the lateral view, check the box where the plumb line should be in relation to the following body landmarks?

Landmark	Anterior	Posterior	Through
Ear			
Tip of the acromion			
Thoracic spine			
Lumbar spine			
Hip			
Knee			
Ankle			

3. View Figure 20-1, indicate in the following table whether the anterior and posterior curves are concave or convex.

Spine Region	Posterior Curve	Anterior Curve
Cervical		
Thoracic		
Lumbar		
Sacral		

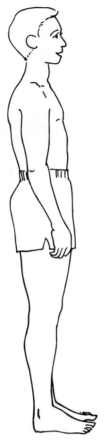

FIGURE 20-1. Anterior and posterior curves.

4. Identify the positions of the pelvis as anterior tilt, neutral, or posterior tilt in Figures 20-2, 20-3 and 20-4.

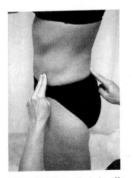

FIGURE 20-2. Pelvic tilt.

_____

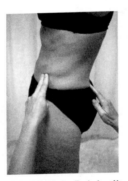

FIGURE 20-3. Pelvic tilt.

_____

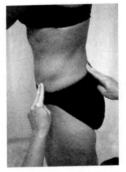

FIGURE 20-4. Pelvic tilt

_____

5. Name the muscle groups that contract concentrically to produce anterior and posterior pelvic tilts.

Position	Muscle Groups
Anterior pelvic tilt	
Posterior pelvic tilt	

6. For a person with a fixed anterior or posterior tilt, identify the muscles that are shortened and those that are lengthened.

Position	Shortened	Lengthened
Anterior pelvic tilt		
Posterior pelvic tilt		

7. In the supine position, a person has an excessive lumbar lordosis. Does this person most likely have _____ an anterior or _____ a posterior pelvic tilt.

8. When standing with good posture, which muscle groups are responsible for maintaining pelvic alignment in the following planes?

Plane	Muscle Groups
Sagittal	
Frontal	
Transverse	

■ ■ ■ Lab Activities

Student's Name _____ Date Due _____

1. Make a chart on the board, list each class member by some identifying code and indicate whether the classmate is right- or left-handed.

   Observe your partner from the posterior view and determine if either the right or left shoulder is higher.

   Enter the information on the chart on the board.

   When all have entered their data, analyze the data for any correlation between shoulder position and hand dominance.

2. Perform an observation of posture. Work in groups of threes.

   A. Suspend a string with a weight (plumb line) from the ceiling.

   B. In all views, position the subject's feet 2–4 inches apart, with the heels even and the toes pointing slightly outward close to the plumb line but not so close that they will touch the plumb line when they sway.

C. Align the plumb line with the feet. In the anterior and posterior views, the plumb line should divide the space between the feet evenly. In the side view the plumb line should be about 2 inches in front of the lateral malleolus.

D. The forms that follow can be used to record your observations.

E. Each member of the group is to be the subject, lead observer, and the assistant observer during this activity.

F. Observe your partner's posture from all views using a plumb line.

G. Do not get too detailed and do not take too long. Some individuals become faint from standing still for a long time due to pooling of blood, work in a timely manner and provide the subject with opportunities to walk around between views.

Anterior View: Deviations from Normal Alignment

Ankles	
Knees	
Hips	
Sternum	
Shoulders	
Face	
Arms	

Posterior View: Deviations from Normal Alignment

Ankles	
Knees	
Hips	
Spinous processes	
Scapula	
Shoulders	
Head	
Arms	

Right Lateral View: Deviations from Normal Alignment

Ankles	
Knees	
Hips	
Lumbar spine	
Thoracic spine	
Acromion process	
Ear	
Top of head	

Left Lateral View: Deviations From Normal Alignment

Ankles	
Knees	
Hips	
Lumbar spine	
Thoracic spine	
Acromion process	
Ear	
Top of head	

3. For a person sitting for long periods, whether in a wheelchair or a desk chair, proper fit of the chair is important. A chair seat that is too wide or short, too high or low interferes with a person's ability to maintain good sitting alignment.

   Position your partner sitting in the ways described here and observe what happens to his or her posture.

   Equipment: various sizes of wheelchairs can be used to make these activities easier. Other types of chairs such as student desk chairs, office chairs, and sofa chairs can be used. For chairs without armrests, place empty chairs on either side with pillows or boxes on the chairs to simulate armrests. Use a footstool, or books of varying thicknesses in front on the floor to simulate footrests.

   A. Have your partner sit in a chair that is much wider than your partner. When using a chair without armrests, place the simulated armrests 6 inches from your partner's hips. Instruct your partner to lean on an armrest. Describe the posture of your partner's spine?

   _____

   B. Have your partner sit in a chair that is narrower than he or she is. Place boxes or pillows to simulate armrests touching your patient. What bony landmark(s) will be under excessive pressure?

   _____

C. With your partner in a sitting position, vary the height of the seat and footrests to achieve the following positions.

1) The hips and knees are at 90° of flexion and the feet are flat on a supporting surface.

2) Adjust a footstool so the hips are in approximately 110° of flexion, the knees are at 90° of flexion, and the feet are flat on a supporting surface.

3) Adjust the height of the seat so that your partner's feet barely reach the floor.

What postural adjustment does your partner make in the second and third positions compared to the first position?

_____

_____

Which bony landmark(s) will be under more pressure in the second and third positions?

_____

_____

■ ■ ■ Post-Lab Questions

Student's Name _____ Date Due _____

After you have completed the Worksheets and Lab Activities, answer the following questions without using your book or notes. When finished, check your answers.

1. List the normal curve of each segment of the spinal column. Describe the posterior side of the curves.

Spinal Segment	Curve
Cervical	
Thoracic	
Lumbar	
Sacral	
Coccyx	

2. For the postural deviations listed in the following table, check the box that is the best view(s) to use to observe the deviation.

Postural Alignment	Anterior View	Posterior View	Lateral View
Coxa vara			
Genu valgus			
Calcaneal varus			
Uneven shoulders			
Genu recurvatum			

3. A posture examination indicates which muscles or structures should be further examined to determine their strength or length. For each of the following postural deviations, list two structures that should be examined and for what purpose.

Postural Alignment	Structure to Examine	Purpose for Examination
Lack of full knee extension		
Anterior pelvic tilt		
Left iliac crest lower than right iliac crest		

Gait

■ ■ ■ An Introduction

The positions of the hip, knee, ankle, and toes have been described for each phase of gait for the Rancho Los Amigos (RLA) approach to gait assessment. These positions are as follows:

INITIAL CONTACT

Hip: 25° Flexion
Knee: 0°
Ankle: 0°
Toes: 0°

LOADING RESPONSE

Hip: 25° Flexion
Knee: 15° Flexion
Ankle: 10° Plantar flexion
Toes: 0°

MIDSTANCE

Hip: 0°
Knee: 0°
Ankle: 5° Dorsiflexion
Toes: 0°

TERMINAL STANCE

Hip: 20° Hyperextension
Knee: 0°
Ankle: 10° Dorsiflexion
Toes: 30° MTP extension

PRESWING

Hip: 0°
Knee: 40° Flexion
Ankle: 20° Plantar flexion
Toes: 60° MTP extension

INITIAL SWING

Hip: 15° Flexion
Knee: 60° Flexion
Ankle: 10° Plantar flexion
Toes: 0°

MIDSWING

Hip: 25° Flexion
Knee: 25° Flexion
Ankle: 0°
Toes: 0°

TERMINAL SWING

Hip: 25° Flexion
Knee: 0°
Ankle: 0°
Toes: 0°

Source: Observational Gait Analysis Handbook. The Pathokinesiology Service and The Physical Therapy Department of Rancho Los Amigos Medical Center, Downey CA, 1993.

■ ■ ■ **Worksheets**

Student's Name _____ Date Due _____

Complete the following questions prior to the lab class.

1. A. A line drawn between successive midpoints of heel strike would reveal what about a person's walking base? _____

   B. What is highest at midstance and lowest at heelstrike? _____

   C. The number of steps taken per minute is called? _____

   D. As the center of gravity shifts from side to side during walking, there are equal amounts of? _____

2. A. In what way are Trendelenburg sign and Trendelenburg gait similar?

   _____

   B. In what way are Trendelenburg sign and Trendelenburg gait different?

   _____

3. Match the following term(s) with the appropriate description:

   _____ Occurs during swing phase

   _____ Body weight shifts allowing one leg to swing

   _____ Body stance phase

   A. Single leg support, midstance

   B. Weight acceptance, heel strike

   C. Leg advancement

4. Match the description with the appropriate period of the gait cycle.

   _____ Occurs during approximately 40% of the gait cycle

   _____ Center of gravity is the lowest point

   _____ Does not occur in walking

   A. Nonsupport

   B. Single-leg support

   C. Double-leg support

5. Match the following descriptions with the appropriate period or point of the gait cycle.

   _____ Between end of toe-off and end of acceleration

   _____ Between end of foot flat and end of midstance

   _____ Between end of midstance and end of heel-off

   _____ The leg swung as far forward as it is going to

   _____ Body weight begins to shift onto stance leg

   _____ Between end of acceleration and end of midswing

   _____ Just before and including when toes leave ground

   _____ Entire foot is in contact with the ground

   A. Initial contact

   B. Foot flat

   C. Midstance

   D. Terminal stance

   E. Preswing

   F. Initial swing

   G. Midswing

   H. Deceleration

6. List in order of occurrence the components of the gait cycle using both traditional terminology and RLA terminology.

Traditional	RLA
STANCE	STANCE
Heel strike	Initial contact
	XX
SWING	SWING

7. Match the following terms and definitions.

_____ Distance between heel strike of one foot and heel strike of the other foot

_____ Side-to-side distance between heels

_____ Distance between heel strike of one foot and heel strike of the same foot

_____ That part of the gait cycle when the foot is in contact with the ground

_____ That part of the gait cycle when the foot is not in contact with the ground

A. Stance phase

B. Stride length

C. Step width

D. Swing phase

E. Step length

8. For each phase of the gait cycle, the amount of range of motion at the hip, knee, and ankle varies. Deviation from the normal range is one of the causes of increased energy cost during walking. For each joint at each phase of the gait cycle, indicate the approximate normal range of motion.

Initial Contact

Joint	ROM
HIP	
KNEE	
ANKLE	
TOES	

Weight Acceptance

Joint	ROM
HIP	
KNEE	
ANKLE	
TOES	

Midstance

Joint	ROM
HIP	
KNEE	
ANKLE	
TOES	

Terminal Stance

Joint	ROM
HIP	
KNEE	
ANKLE	
TOES	

Preswing

Joint	ROM
HIP	
KNEE	
ANKLE	
TOES	

Initial Swing

Joint	ROM
HIP	
KNEE	
ANKLE	
TOES	

Midswing

Joint	ROM
HIP	
KNEE	
ANKLE	
TOES	

Terminal Swing

Joint	ROM
HIP	
KNEE	
ANKLE	
TOES	

9. Joint movement during gait is produced by muscle contractions, gravity and joint response in a closed kinetic chain. Determining the direction of joint movement, within a phase and from one phase of gait to the next, is necessary to analyze which muscles are working and what type of contraction a muscle is performing. For each phase of the gait cycle indicate:

A. The position (or motion) that is occurring at each joint; and

B. Briefly describe what is happening. Examples are: unchanged; slight flexion from full extension; and increasing dorsiflexion.

Initial Contact (from Terminal Swing)

Joint	Position	Describe
HIP		
KNEE		
ANKLE		

Loading Response (from Initial Contact)

Joint	Position	Describe
HIP		
KNEE		
ANKLE		

Midstance (from Loading Response)

Joint	Position	Describe
HIP		
KNEE		
ANKLE		

Terminal Stance (from Midstance)

Joint	Position	Describe
HIP		
KNEE		
ANKLE		

Preswing (from Terminal Stance)

Joint	Position	Describe
HIP		
KNEE		
ANKLE		

Initial Swing (from Preswing)

Joint	Position	Describe
HIP		
KNEE		
ANKLE		

Midswing (from Initial Swing)

Joint	Position	Describe
HIP		
KNEE		
ANKLE		

Terminal Swing (from Midswing)

Joint	Position	Describe
HIP		
KNEE		
ANKLE		

■ ■ ■ Lab Activities

Student's Name _____ Date Due _____

1. As a class, demonstrate each phase of the gait cycle.

2. Step length, stride length, and step width can be measured using simple methods. One method is:

   A. Tape about a 10-foot length of absorbent paper on the floor with a chair placed at one end.

   B. The subject dips the bottoms of bare feet in water and walks with a normal gait and cadence. One observer records the time to walk from the first heel strike to the last heel strike on the paper.

   C. Place a mark at, and label, each heel strike as either right or left foot.

   D. Measure the distances between heel strikes of the same foot, heel strikes of opposite feet, and the width between heel strikes of opposite feet.

   E. Count the number of strides and use the time walked to determine the speed of the gait.

3. Observe the gait of your partners from the front, side, and back. This is most easily done using a treadmill. If one is not available, arrange an area large enough so the subject is able to walk at normal speed and the observers have sufficient room to observe and move as needed to observe from the front, back and each side. When observing from the side, the observers walk sideways to be able to observe the subject directly as the subject walks.

   A. Initial observations should be of the "whole person" as the individual walks. Note speed and any unusual gait patterns.

   B. Observe each joint through the full cycle of gait, identifying the phase.

C. Observe each joint through the full cycle to determine the ROM. Make note of any ROM at any joint that is not normal. On the following form, indicate the phase of the gait cycle and if the ROM is less than normal (−), or greater than normal (+), or normal (N).

Initial Contact

Joint	ROM
HIP	
KNEE	
ANKLE	
TOES	

Loading Response

Joint	ROM
HIP	
KNEE	
ANKLE	
TOES	

Midstance

Joint	ROM
HIP	
KNEE	
ANKLE	
TOES	

Terminal Stance

Joint	ROM
HIP	
KNEE	
ANKLE	
TOES	

Preswing

Joint	ROM
HIP	
KNEE	
ANKLE	
TOES	

Initial Swing

Joint	ROM
HIP	
KNEE	
ANKLE	
TOES	

Midswing

Joint	ROM
HIP	
KNEE	
ANKLE	
TOES	

Terminal Swing

Joint	ROM
HIP	
KNEE	
ANKLE	
TOES	

4. Being able to identify typical gait deviations is important. Imitating gait deviations is one way to learn to identify atypical gait patterns and the energy requirements that result. Imitate the following gait deviations and observe your partner imitating those gait deviations.

General Cause of Abnormal Gait	Description of Resulting Abnormal Gait
Gluteus maximus weakness	Compensated by: Quickly shift the trunk posteriorly at heel strike (initial contact) on the side of the weak gluteus maximus so COG is posterior to axis of hip joint.
Gluteus medius weakness	Compensated by: Shift the trunk over the side of the weak gluteus medius during stance.
Quadriceps weakness	Compensated by: At heel strike (initial contact and loading response) on the side of the weakness, lean your body forward so COG is anterior to axis of knee joint. Another method is to use the ipsilateral hand to hold the knee in extension during stance.
Hamstring weakness	Uncompensated: Excessive or fast extension of the knee during deceleration (terminal swing).
Ankle dorsiflexor weakness	Uncompensated: Toes strike ground first instead of the heel = equinnus gait. Strength permits heel strike (initial contact) to occur but not controlled movement to foot flat (loading response) resulting in foot slap. During swing phase the ankle remains in plantar flexion = drop foot. Compensated by excessive hip flexion = steppage gait.
Triceps surae group weakness	Uncompensated: No heel rise or push-off resulting in a shortened step length on the unaffected side.
Diffuse weakness of many muscle groups	Compensated by: Waddling gait; shoulders posterior to hips and lateral shift to weight-bearing side. Little pelvic motion. To advance a leg, the entire side of the body swings forward. Excessive hip flexion may be needed because of ankle dorsiflexor weakness.
Hip flexion contracture	Compensated by: During stance on the involved side, the trunk leans forward.
Fused hip	Compensated by: Increased motion of the lumbar spine and pelvis.
Knee flexion contracture	Excessive dorsiflexion during midstance and an early heel rise during push-off (terminal stance). Short step length on unaffected side.
Knee fused in extension	Compensated by: 1. Toe rise of uninvolved side during stance to allow involved side to clear during midswing = vaulting gait. 2. Hip hike on the involved side during swing. 3. Swing leg out to side = circumducted gait.

(Continued...)

General Cause of Abnormal Gait	Description of Resulting Abnormal Gait
Triceps surae contracture: Ankle in plantarflexion	Uncompensated: Knee forced into excessive extension during midstance; unable to progress tibia over foot from midstance on.
Ankle fusion: Triple arthrodesis	Uncompensated: Loss of ankle pronation and supination= makes walking on uneven surfaces difficult; limited ankle dorsiflexion and plantarflexion; short stride length.
Ataxic gait	Uncompensated: Poor balance, uneven, jerky, exaggerated movements. Compensated by: Wide base of support.
Scissors gait	Uncompensated: Excessive adduction and lateral body shift during swing phase; narrow base.
Crouch gait	Uncompensated: Increased lumbar lordosis; anterior pelvic tilt; excessive hip flexion, adduction and medial rotation; excessive knee flexion; ankles plantar flexed. Compensated by: Excessive arm movement.
Antalgic gait	Compensated by: Short stance phase on involved side results in rapid and short step length of the uninvolved side. May alter arm swing.

5. In a group, observe what happens to the components of gait as an individual varies cadence from very slow to very fast (do not run). Describe the changes you observe.

_____

_____

6. In a group, observe what happens to the components of gait when an individual uses an assistive device such as a cane, walker, and sling on one arm. Describe how the gait changes in each situation.

Cane: _____

Walker: _____

Sling: _____

■ ■ ■ Post-Lab Questions

Student's Name _____ Date Due _____

After you have completed the Worksheets and Lab Activities, answer the following questions without using your book or notes. When finished, check your answers.

1. Identify the following descriptions of gait phases by giving the traditional terminology and the RLA terminology.

Description of Gait Phase	Traditional Terminology	Rancho Los Amigos Terminology
Body weight shock is absorbed		
Hip at maximum flexion		
Hip is hyperextended and knee is starting to flex		
The foot strikes the ground		
Period of single limb support		
Leg behind body and moving forward		
Dorsiflexors contract eccentrically		
Body passes over weight-bearing leg		
Hamstrings contract eccentrically		
Toes are in extreme hyperextension		

2. Indicate the direction of movement (flexing or extending) at the joints listed in the following phases of gait.

   A. Heel strike to foot flat—initial contact to loading response

   Knee: _____

   Ankle: _____

   B. Foot flat to midstance—loading response to midstance

   Hip: _____

   Ankle: _____

   C. Heel-off to toe-off—terminal stance to initial swing

   Knee: _____

   Ankle: _____

   D. Acceleration to midswing—initial swing to midswing

   Hip: _____

   Knee: _____

3. In which phases of gait do the following motions occur?

   A. Hip flexion: _____

   B. Knee extension: _____

   C. Ankle dorsiflexion: _____